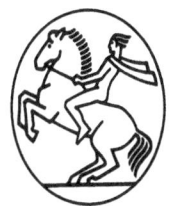

Gunnar B. J. Andersson
and Thomas W. McNeill

Lumbar Spine Syndromes
Evaluation and Treatment

Springer-Verlag Wien New York

Gunnar B. J. Andersson, M.D., Ph.D.
Thomas W. McNeill, M.D.

Department of Orthopedic Surgery
Rush-Presbyterian-St. Luke's Medical Hospital
Chicago, Illinois, U.S.A.

With 108 Figures

Library of Congress Cataloging-in-Publication Data: Andersson, Gunnar, 1942–; Lumbar spine syndromes: evaluation and treatment / Gunnar B.J. Andersson and Thomas W. McNeill. VII, 215 p. 16.3 × 24.3 cm. Includes bibliographies and index. ISBN-13: 978-3-7091-8983-2   1. Backache. I. McNeill, Thomas W., 1936–. II. Title. [DNLM: 1. Backache–diagnosis. 2. Backache–therapy. WE 755 A 552 L] RD 771.B 217 A 53 1988; 617'. 56–dc 19; CIP 88-24942

ISBN-13: 978-3-7091-8983-2   e-ISBN-13: 978-3-7091-8981-8
DOI: 10.1007/978-3-7091-8981-8

Preface

The question facing anyone contemplating a book on low back pain is: Why write another book? It is certainly true that there are many books on this topic addressing a wide variety of audiences. Some books are all inclusive and scholarly in nature, others are personal descriptions of diagnostic and treatment philosophies. This book is a combination of these two extremes. It represents our views on the low back problem, supported by scientific data. Most aspects on back pain presented in this book can be found in other texts. The organization of the material is unique, however.

Our approach is to start by listening to and looking at the patient. It becomes apparent, then, that patients can be classified into one of the syndromes described in chapters 4 through 13. We believe that this syndrome classification, which is quite simple to make clinically, will allow you to diagnose and treat your patients more effectively. To set the stage for the syndrome chapters the first three chapters of the book are generic to the remaining chapters. They reviewe the epidemiology, pathology, biomechanics, etiologic theory, diagnostic methods, and treatment modalities applicable to the low back syndromes. They should be read before the syndrome chapters. At the end of the book you will find four chapters that are specific to disease entities. They were included to allow a separate discussion of this small, but important, group of diseases with symptoms and signs common to the lumbar spinal syndromes, but with specific diagnostic requirements, treatment and prognosis.

This book is not intended for the super specialist. Rather, it should be helpful to physicians, of different specialities, who deal with back pain patients as part of their practices, and to the medical resident who wishes to understand the principles of back pain management.

Many have supported our efforts. In particular we express our gratitude to Robert N. Hensinger, M.D., who wrote the chapter on back pain in children. Glen D. Dobben, M.D., provided invaluable assistance in writing the section on imaging techniques. Ms. Judith Weik did the artwork expertly with superb artistic finesse. Mrs. Dorothy Bell typed, retyped and retyped cheerfully and carefully.

Finally we wish to thank our families who supported us. The time it took to complete our effort cannot be replaced.

G. B. J. Andersson and T. W. McNeill

Contents

1 Introduction

Historical perspective

The species of sciatica are various, according to the various parts in which the pain is felt; and altho' as hitherto, physicians have not discriminated between them so accurately as they ought ...
Diminicus Contunnius, 1775

Low back pain, with or without sciatica, is one of the most common complaints presenting to a physician. The causes of these complaints are numerous and include pathological changes in several different tissues, structures and organs. To the physician in the past low back pain, as a symptom of systemic disease was more important than back pain originating from pathological changes of the spinal structures per se. Low back pain as an independent issue did not become clinically important until the 1930's. At that time a combination of changes in the political, social and medical arena gave the complaint of low back pain new importance. Medical interest rose rapidly after Mixter and Barr (1934) "rediscovered" the herniated intervertebral disc and offered the possibility of a surgical "cure" for some varieties of this condition. At the same time there was the rapid political acceptance of worker's compensation laws in the United States, Canada, and Europe. This new social legislation provided compensation for injuries sustained on the job or as a result of the job. Complaining of low back pain then became more meaningful, and accepted. The next link in the chain of events leading up to the current situation was the acceptance of the concept that the likely cause of most low back pain is an injury, which either caused the painful episode directly or, if pain was preexisting, aggravated it. Considerable effort has been expended in laboratories throughout the world to explain the pathological changes in and the mechanisms of these "injuries". These efforts have had little effect on the problem of low back pain, however, and in fact the incidence has increased in recent years increasing the cost of low back pain to both industry and to society as a whole (Fig. 1).

In the 1850's Virchow and Luschka described the protruded intervertebral disc. Luschka's illustrations of a prolapse of the intervertebral disc would be difficult to improve upon today; and, he speculated correctly that

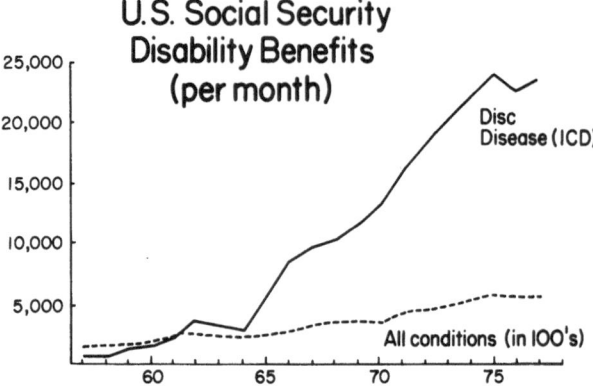

Fig. 1. Annual statistics for U.S. Social Security Disability Insurance. Awards for permanent and total disability. (Adapted from Waddell, 1987)

the disc herniation might produce cord compression. In 1911 Middleton and Teacher from Glasgow described a patient who had developed paraplegia as a result of herniation of an intervertebral disc. They also did an ad hoc experiment designed to demonstrate that the mechanism of injury (a lifting overload) could produce a discal hernia. At about the same time in Boston, Goldthwait (1911) described a patient who had developed paraplegia following unsuccessful treatment for "sacro-iliac sprain". In 1929 Andrae examined 368 spines and found 56 posterior disc herniations. In 1934 Mixter and Barr described the clinical syndrome of rupture of the lumbar intervertebral disc and its successful surgical treatment. A 1985 publication by Frymoyer and Doneghy has given us a fifty year follow-up examination of Mixter and Barr's first patient. In 1952 Hirsch and Schajowitz summarized the evidence implicating the disc as a source of low back pain and added an exhaustive pathologic analysis of the changes found in the annulus fibrosis. The intervertebral disc remains implicated as one of the commonest "causes" of lower back pain. It gets increasingly clear, however, that the disc is not the only source of pain, and, in fact, may not even be the most important.

The facet joints (apophyseal joints) have also attracted significant attention over the years. Goldthwait (1911) and Putti (1927) both considered these joints to be sources of back pain and sciatica, and Ghormley (1933) coined the phrase "facet syndrome". More recently these joints have again attracted more attention and diagnostic tests and specific treatment has been suggested for this syndrome (Rees, 1971; Shealy, 1974; Mooney and Robertson, 1976; Farfan, 1985).

The muscles of the back as well as the ligamentous structures have always been considered as possible sources of pain, but there is little scientific support that this is in fact the case. Kellgren (1938, 1939) stimulated muscle,

ligaments and joints mechanically and chemically and found that the resulting pain was rather constant in its distribution for any given structure in any
given individual. Stimulation of very deep structures resulted in pain with
segmental distribution.

Incidence, prevalence, and costs

The importance of low back disorders in the industrial world cannot be
overstated. About 60–80% of the population is affected by low back pain at
sometime during their lives. In the United States, impairments of the back
and spine are the chronic conditions most frequently causing limitations in
activities in persons under 40 years of age. Low back pain is also the diagnosis
in about 10% of all chronic health conditions. The estimated prevalence of
self-reported back symptoms in the U.S. is about 17%, indicating that more
than 30,000,000 Americans have back pain. It has also been estimated that
about 1% of all adults in the U.S. have a prolapsed disc at any one point in
time (Gracier et al., 1984). Similar data emerges from the United Kingdom,
where surveys have shown that 25% of all working men are affected by low
back disorders each year and that one out of 25 workers change their jobs
because of their back's condition (Pope et al., 1984). On any one day, 0.5%
of the work force in Great Britain has been chronically disabled for more
than six months by a back problem (Wood and Badley, 1980).

Swedish statistics show that low back pain is responsible for an average
of 12% of all sickness-absence stay and that the average sickness-absence
period is about 30 days. While 30% of all sickness-absence periods are
shorter than one week, 9% last for 3 months or longer.

Cross-sectional studies from the United States, Scandinavia, Israel and
the Netherlands all report life-time incidence rates at similar levels, suggesting that the problem of low back pain is common to all industrial countries
(Table 1). Operations for back pain, however, are more common in the
United States than elsewhere. Thus, about 115,000 laminectomies as well as
34,000 other lumbar spine operations are performed in the U.S. each year.

Although it is difficult to determine the costs of the low back problem
precisely, it has been estimated that in the United States the direct cost is at
least $16,000,000,000 per year. This figure increases dramatically when indi-
rect costs are included.

The first episodes of low back pain most often occur in people in their 20's
and 30's. Back pain in men seems to peak around age 40, while in women
there is a further dramatic increase from age 50 to age 60 (Biering-Sorensen,
1982). This could be due to osteoporosis playing an increasingly important
role in women with advancing age. Males and females are otherwise equally
affected, but operations for disc hernias are twice as frequent in men as in

Table 1. Life-time incidence and prevalence rates reported in cross-sectional studies

Study	Life-time incidence %	Prevalence	N	Sex
Biering-Sorensen (1982)	62.6	12.0	449	M
	61.4	15.2	479	F
Frymoyer et al. (1983)	69.9		1221	M
Svensson/Andersson (1982)	61.0	31	716	M
(1988)	66.0	35	1760	F
Valkenburg/Haanen (1982)	51.4	22.2	3091	M
	57.8	30.2	3493	F

women. The mean age for disc hernia operations is about 42 years in both men and women.

Although much work has been devoted to identifying individual risk factors, few hold up to scientific scrutiny (Andersson, 1981). Data on the importance of anthropometric factors and postural deformities are conflicting and do not indicate strong relationships to low back. The same is true for spine mobility, muscle strength, and physical fitness. Radiographic factors are also poor predictors of risk of low back pain as discussed in Chap. 2. Smoking appears to be a habit increasing the risk of low back pain and there are also studies indicating that social factors are important (Pope et al., 1984; Frymoyer, 1988).

Work-related risk factors include repetitive lifting, particularly in forward bent and twisting positions, exposure to vibration and predominantly static work posture (Pope et al., 1984; Andersson, 1981). The importance of work factors in the context of low back pain is obvious from a report published by the National Institute for Occupational Safety and Health in 1981. The report states that overexertion is claimed as a cause of low back pain by over 60% of low back patients and that low back "injuries" occur to about 500,000 workers per year. Most of these "injuries", fortunately, heal in a short period of time. The long lasting (chronic) low back "injuries", however, are very costly. Snook (1980) found that 25% of these cases accounted for 90% of the costs, while Spengler et al. (1986) found that 10% of back injuries accounted for nearly 80% of the total costs.

The natural history of low back pain and sciatica

Low back pain and sciatica are generally self-limiting conditions. Epidemiologic studies indicate a recovery rate of 70% in three weeks and of 90% in

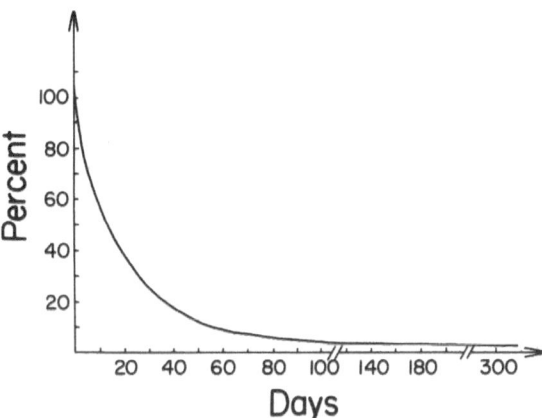

Fig. 2. Recovery rate for patients who report sick from back conditions. (Adapted from Andersson et al., 1983)

6–12 weeks (Andersson et al., 1983; Frymoyer, 1988) (Fig. 2). The recovery rate in sciatica is slower than in low back pain, but 50 percent of patients with sciatica do recover within a month (Fig. 3 a, b). Unfortunately low back pain is recurrent in nature with an increased risk of recurrence in sciatica and severe back disease (Biering-Sorensen, 1983).

Functional anatomy and biomechanics

The spine has three mechanical functions; to support the trunk; to protect the spinal cord and nerve roots; and to allow motion of the trunk and head. To accomplish these functions a rather complex structure has evolved. In the following, a brief review of the functional anatomy and biomechanics of the spine is given, to the purpose of introduction rather than completeness. For further reading please refer to, for example, White and Panjabi (1978), Andersson (1982), Schultz (1982), and Pope et al. (1982).

The vertebral column

The vertebral column consists of 33 vertebrae, of which, in the adult, nine are fused together for form the sacrum and coccyx. The sacrum is attached to the pelvis such that only little motion occurs. The 24 mobile vertebrae are divided into 5 lumbar, 12 thoracic and 7 cervical (Fig. 4). These are joined together by the intervertebral discs, the intervertebral joints, and several ligaments. When discussing the spinal structures, it is useful to consider first the whole of the spine, and then the so-called *motion segment*, which is defined as two adjacent vertebrae, the intervening disc, and the associated ligamentous

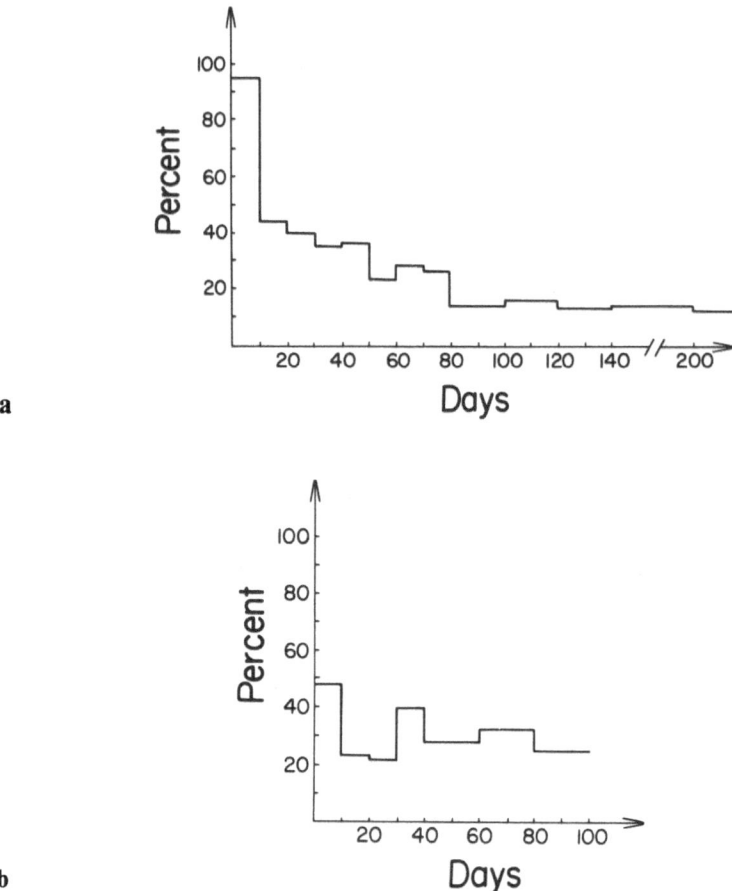

a

b

Fig. 3. Percent of patients returning to work at 10 day intervals of those who were absent during the previous interval: **a** all back pain, **b** sciatica. (Adapted from Andersson et al., 1983)

structures (Figs. 5 and 6). The motion segment can be considered as a functional unit, a building block, and is the structure on which most experimental studies have been carried out in vitro. From a physiological point of view, the in vivo motion segment also includes the associated nerves and muscles (Fig. 7).

The vertebral column is straight in the antero-posterior view and curved in the lateral view. There is a cervical lordosis, a thoracic kyphosis, and a lumbar lordosis (Fig. 4). This shape results from the shapes of the vertebrae and discs, their height being greater anteriorly than posteriorly, and is influenced by the ribcage and the inclination of the sacral end-plate. The intervertebral discs constitute about 25 per cent of the height of the vertebral column, more in the lumbar and cervical regions and less in the thoracic.

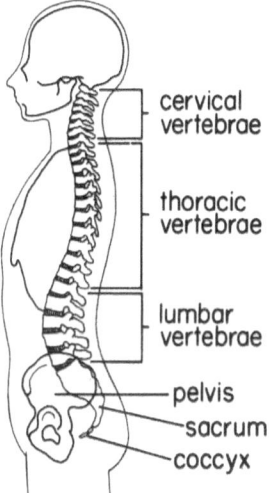

Fig. 4. The different parts of the spine

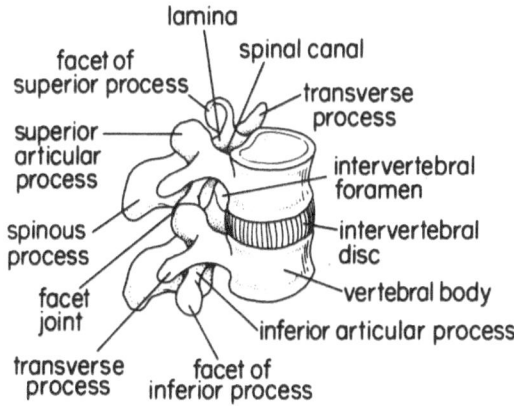

Fig. 5. The bony elements and disc of a motion segment. (Adapted from Fine, 1985)

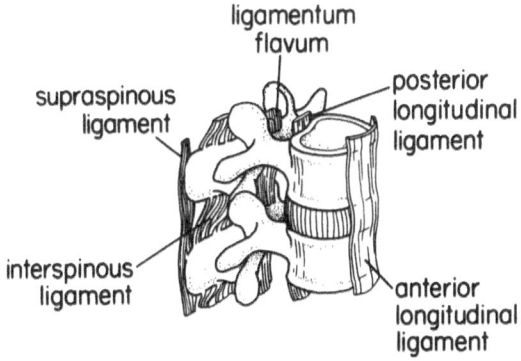

Fig. 6. The ligaments of a motion segment. Lateral view. (Adapted from Fine, 1985)

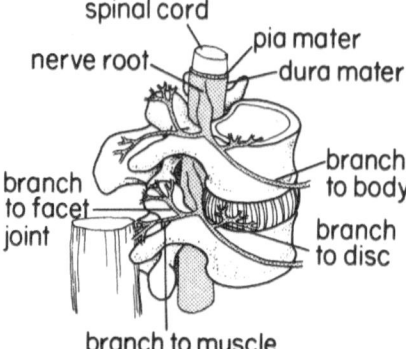

Fig. 7. The nervous structures of a motion segment. (Adapted from Fine, 1985)

There is large individual variation in the shape of vertebrae and discs and thus in the curvatures of the spine. The variation in shape of the vertebral column is further emphasized by a 40 degree variation in the inclination of the sacral end-plate. This inclination is of mechanical importance as the shear stress on the lumbosacral articulation increases with increasing vertical incli- nation of the sacral end-plate. The shape of the spine is functionally advan- tageous allowing for considerable energy absorption and thus protecting the spine from impacts and vibrations.

When looking at a cross-section of the spine at a lumbar vertebral level, the bony parts and soft tissues can be divided into *anterior* and *posterior elements* (Fig. 8). The dividing line is just behind the vertebral body, leaving anteriorly the body, the disc, and the anterior and posterior longitudinal ligaments. Posteriorly lie the neural arch with its processes, the intervertebral joints (also named apophyseal joints and facet joints), and the different

POSTERIOR ELEMENTS

ANTERIOR ELEMENTS

Fig. 8. The vertebral column can be divided into anterior and posterior elements

ligaments attached to the bony structures. This division is not merely anatomical, but has a functional (mechanical) purpose. The anterior elements provide the major support of the column and absorb various impacts; the posterior structures control the patterns of motion. Both elements protect the spinal cord, which lies posterior to the vertebral body surrounded by the neural arch.

The ligaments

The seven ligaments of the spine can be divided into three systems. A *longitudinal* system (a), includes the anterior and posterior longitudinal ligaments and the supraspinous ligaments, a *segmental* system (b), includes the interspinous, intertransverse ligaments and the ligamentae flava (yellow ligaments), and an *articular* or *capsular* system (c), includes the ligaments of the apophyseal joints (Fig. 9). The ligaments aid in the control of motion but offer only limited stability to the spine, which in fact when stripped of muscles and loaded in the laboratory buckles at loads as low as 40 Newtons (4 kg).

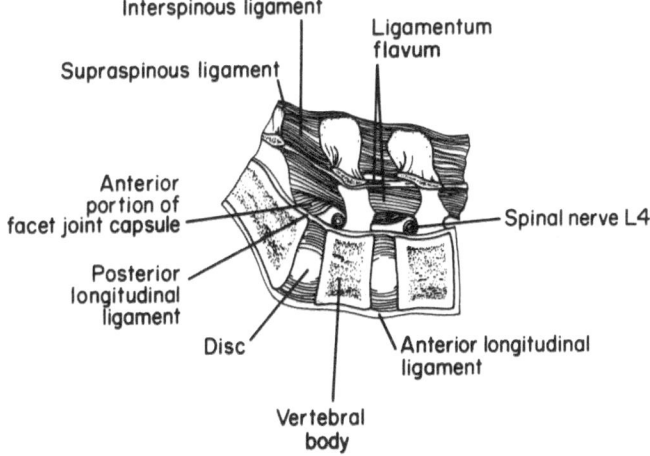

Fig. 9. The ligaments of the spine viewed in a sagittal section. (Adapted from Hoppenfeld, 1976)

The motion segment

Loads applied to a motion segment in vitro, in a way simulate loading occuring in vivo and therefore give insight into the response of the tissues to such loads (i.e., deformation and failure). Compressive load means that a downward force is applied perpendicular to the upper vertebra, tension is when the motion segment is pulled apart, twisting when rotation is applied and shear loading when the upper vertebra is translated on the lower (or the opposite). In life loading will almost always be a combination of these different basic types of load applications.

When a compressive load is applied to a motion segment failure occurs first in the end-plate, then in the vertebral bodies and only thereafter in the disc proper. The moment-rotation and force-deformation properties of the motion segments in different modes of loading are now also available from the literature (Schultz, 1982). They have been found to vary greatly between individuals, more so than between age-groups. They are also affected by degeneration, but again to a lesser degree than the inter-individual variation.

The intervertebral disc

The disc is formed by two histologically, chemically and mechanically distinct structures; the nucleus, an incompressible watery gel, and the annulus, in which fibrous lamellae are arranged differently from layer to layer (Fig. 10). The different properties of the two parts of the disc produce its load-bearing characteristics. Because of its high water content the nucleus has nearly hydrostatic properties. When the disc is loaded the nucleus deforms and transfers the force in all directions. The fiber arrangement of the annulus is well adapted to accept axial tensile stresses which decreases the risk of structural failure.

The disc is separated from the vertebral bodies by hyaline cartilage end-plates. These influence the nutrition to the disc, which because of its lack of

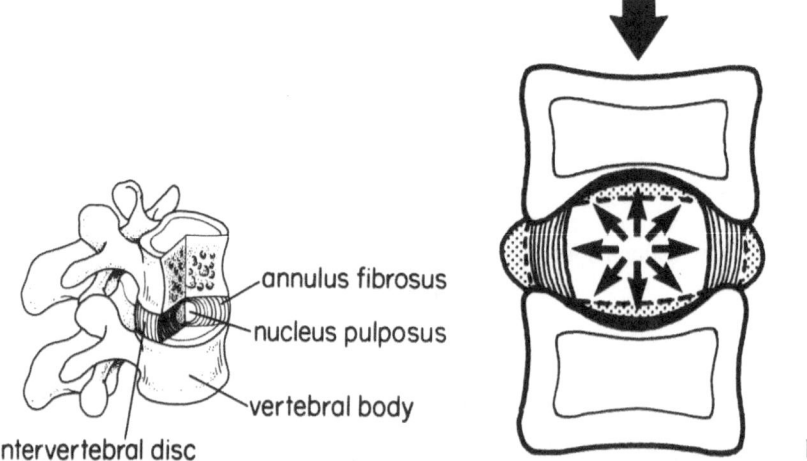

a   intervertebral disc   b

Fig. 10. The disc consists of a centrally located nucleus fibrosus surrounded by the fibers of the annulus fibrosus. **a** Longitudinal section, **b** when loaded the disc nucleus distributes the load in all directions. (Adapted from Fine, 1985)

vascular tissue occurs by diffusion only. The diffusion of fluid and nutrients into the disc is influenced by mechanical factors. When the load on the disc increases there is an outflow of fluid, when it decreases there is a fluid influx. This explains why we are taller immediately after getting up in the morning and then become a centimeter or so shorter over the day.

The response of the disc to compression has been studied extensively. These studies show that the disc is quite flexible at low loads, but provides increasing resistance to load at high loads. Disc herniations have not been produced by compression alone, although after fracture of the end-plate, disc material has been found to spread into the vertebral bodies. Adams and Hutton (1985) produced disc hernias when the posterior elements were first removed, and then a combination of flexion and compression was applied. Farfan (1973) has found that the disc is particularly at risk when subjected to bending and rotation and has put forward the hypothesis that torsion is the main reason for disc failure.

The muscles

The muscles of the back can be divided into antero-lateral prevertebral muscles, deep postvertebral muscles, and superficial covering back muscles. In addition, anterior and lateral abdominal muscles, and also the gluteal muscles aid in the control of trunk motion and in support of the ligamentous spine (Fig. 11). The supportive role is important because without muscles the spine is unstable. The antero-lateral muscles in the lumbar region support the vertebral column (psoas major and minor), and act as lateral flexors (quadratus lumborum). The deep postvertebral muscles are often divided into a transversospinal group and a sacrospinal group, the erector spinae muscles (ESM) (MacIntosh and Bogduk, 1987). The transversospinal muscles are short muscles, spanning one or a few motion segment, close to the vertebral

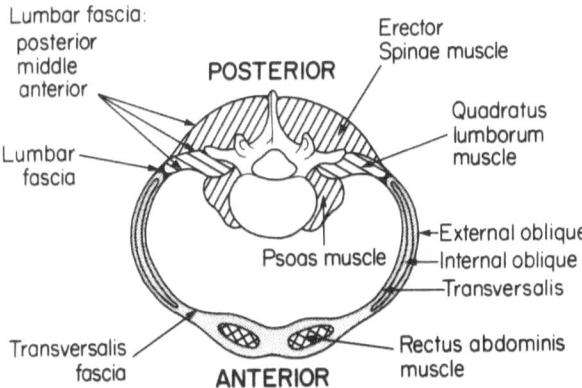

Fig. 11. A cross-section of the trunk at the L3 level

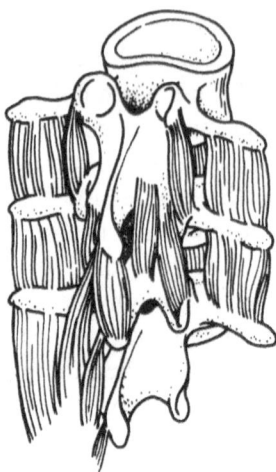

Fig. 12. The transversospinal muscles of the back. (Adapted from Fine, 1985)

column (Fig. 12). The sacrospinal muscles, on the other hand, are long muscles lateral to the vertebral column (Fig. 13). The functions of these groups of muscles vary, depending on direction of movement and external loading. They are all active, but to a different degree, in extension, flexion, rotation, and lateral bending of the spine. Superficial back muscles cover the ESM almost completely except in the lumbar region where they insert into the thoraco-lumbar fascia which extends over the ESM. The superficial muscle have an important supportive role and major functions in movements of the trunk during physical activities.

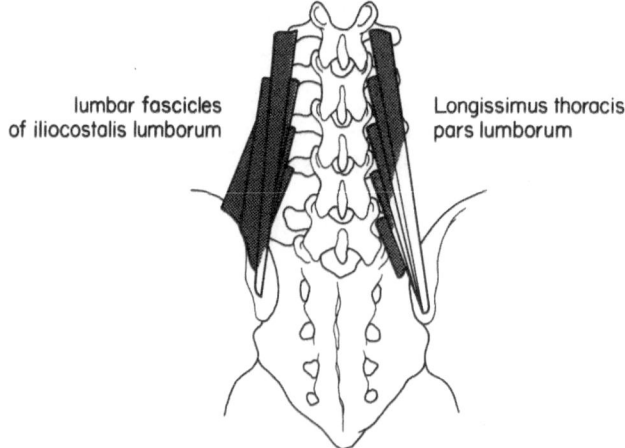

Fig. 13. The lumbar parts of the iliocostalis lumborum and longissimus muscles. (Adapted from MacIntosh and Bogduk, 1986)

The intervertebral joints

The intervertebral joints (apophyseal joints or facet joints) are the only synovial joints of the spine (Fig. 14). One of the primary functions of the lumbar facet joints is to protect the disc from excessive torsion which can lead to disc failure. A second function is to carry compressive loads, which is shared between the facet joints and the disc. These joints have also a significant stabilizing effect on the motion segment in flexion and extension. When the facet joints are removed experimentally, significantly more angular displacement occurs in response to given loads (Schultz, 1982).

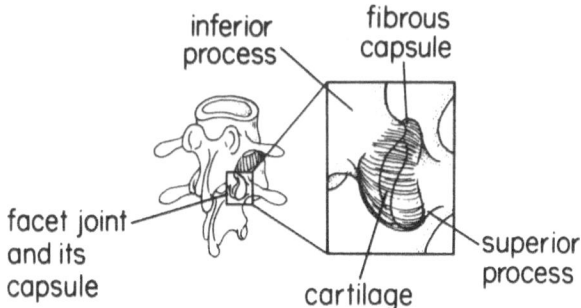

Fig. 14. The facet joint (apophyseal joint). (Adapted from Fine, 1985)

The vertebral bodies

The vertebral bodies consist of a shell of cortical bone enclosing a meshwork of cancellous bone. The effect of a significant trauma to the vertebral body is a fracture. The failure force has been reported to be of the order of 6000 N or less (Fig. 15), decreasing with increasing age. Large fractures can be seen radiographically. Histological studies have shown that in addition there are fractures of the cancellous bone trabeculae, not detectable on radiograms. These "microfractures" increase in number with the bone mineral content of the vertebrae decreasing.

The neural arch

The neural (vertebral) arch provides the lateral and posterior bony perimeters of the neural canal. It carries on both sides articular processes which divide the arch into anterior parts, called pedicles, and posterior parts, called laminae. Directly posterior is the spinous process, and on both sides, attached to the arch, the transverse processes. The articular processes carry the articular facets of the facet joints. There are two such facets, called the superior and inferior (articulating superiorly and inferiorly), and these are connected

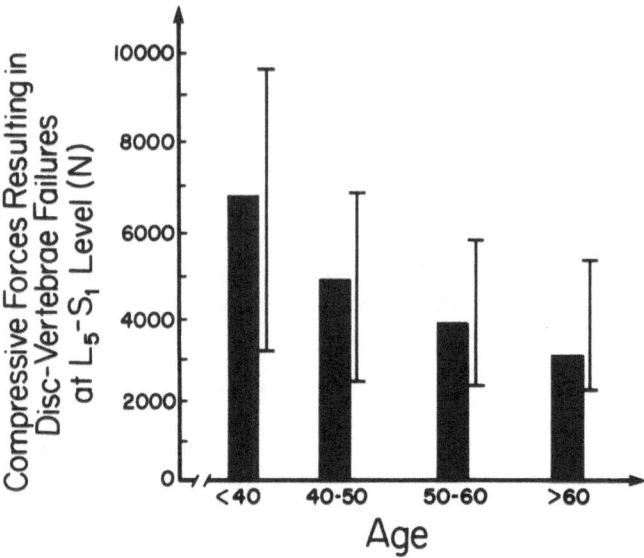

Fig. 15. Disc compression failures by age (means and range). (Adapted from NIOSH, 1982)

through the so-called vertebral isthmus or pars interarticularis. When the isthmus is fractured or destroyed, this is the lesion called spondylolysis. When the lesion allows one vertebral segment to slip forward on another a step deformity occurs, which is called spondylolisthesis.

The spinal cord and nerve roots

The change in the length of the spinal canal occuring with motion of the spine has a major influence on the cord and nerve roots. The cord adapts to the length changes of the canal. This is possible without causing undue tension because, in the neutral position, the cord is folded. Thus, in flexion the cord unfolds much like an accordion before tension occurs, while in extension it folds further before compression takes place. This unfolding and folding mechanism has been found to prevail during 70 to 75 per cent of a full range of flexion-extension movement. The nerve roots follow the spinal cord, but do not fold and unfold. This results in nerve root tension in flexion and during leg raising.

Motion of the spine

The two principal types of motion, translation and rotation, are normally coupled in the spine, i.e., to a certain degree both types of motion occur simultaneously. For example, in a flexion movement each vertebra rotates in the sagittal plane, and at the same time it translates in the same plane.

Flexion and extension are the main modes of motion in the cervical region but considerable axial rotation and lateral bending is also possible. While the main part of the flexion-extension movement and lateral bending occurs in the mid-cervical region, axial rotation occurs primarily in the upper part of the cervical spine. In the thoracic region there is generally little motion; it is stabilized by the ribcage. The lumbar spine permits considerable lateral bending in the mid-portion, while flexion-extension is greatest in the lumbo-sacral motion segment. Rotation is minimal in the lumbar region because of the orientation of the facet joints.

The greater mobility in the cervical and lumbar regions increases the stresses on the tissues there. It is therefore not surprising that most clinical complaints stem from these parts of the spine.

Stability

The stability of the lumbar spine is largely provided by the anterior elements. The facet joints play an additional important role, stabilizing primarily in axial rotation. Due to the large muscle mass surrounding the lumbar spine significant active stability is also present. White and Panjabi (1978) have discussed in detail the concept of clinical instability, defined as the ability of the spine to limit displacement under physiological load. Any disruption of the different spine structures will decrease the clinical stability, but in varying proportions. When the anterior elements are totally destroyed, for example through a burst fracture or a tumor, there is gross instability, while compression fractures of the vertebral bodies may in fact increase the strength of the vertebral body and provide an increased stability. In the first instance, therefore, instability must be dealt with in the treatment, while patients with compression type fractures can be mobilized immediately. This interesting phenomenon has to do with the orientation of the bone trabeculae which is mainly longitudinal. When compressed the trabeculae are forced into each other much like in pushing one hairbrush into another one.

Loads on the spine in vivo

Knowledge of the loads that act on the component structures of the spine in different physical activities is useful to relate those activities to spine injury, and to institute and evaluate preventive measures. There are no methods available at the present time to measure directly in vivo loads on all spinal structures. The loads can be measured indirectly, however, and can also be evaluated through biomechanical model analysis. The indirect load measures include measurements of pressures in discs and in the abdominal cavity as well as measurement of back muscle activities. The measurements obtained shed limited light on the injury and failure mechanisms occurring. It is obviously not acceptable to load a spine in vivo until it fails. Nevertheless, the measurements do provide some insight into the possible dangers of certain activities and load situations allowing inference to unacceptable loads.

Disc pressure measurement

The disc pressure method was developed by Nachemson (1960), who showed that the disc nucleus behaved hydrostatically. Following measurements in vitro several studies have been performed in vivo using a pressure transducer attached to the tip of a needle which is inserted into the disc. The pressure has been found to increase linearly with an increase in trunk moment; for example, when bending forward or carrying and lifting loads. The measurements show that the L3 disc in daily activities often experiences loads three to four times the body weight above that level (Table 2).

Table 2. Approximate loads in Newton (N) on the L 3 disc in a 70 kg individual as calculated from disc pressure measurements. (Adapted from Nachemson, 1981)

Activity	Load (N)
Standing	500
Sitting, unsupported	700
Sitting, well supported	400
Supine	250
Semi-Fowler position (supine)	100
Standing/Coughing	700
Forward bending 40°	1000
Lifting 100 N	1700
Holding 50 N arms extended	1900
Sitting office chair	500
Raising, no armrests	1000

Intra-abdominal pressure measurement

Intra-abdominal (intragastric) pressure measurements have also been used as indicators of the load on the spine. The idea that pressures within the trunk reflect the load on the spine is based on the hypothesis that the pressure in the trunk cavities supports the vertebral column, particularly when the trunk

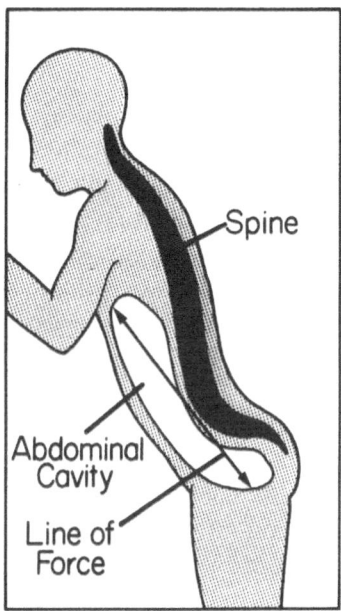

Fig. 16. The effect of the intraabdominal pressure

is flexed (Fig. 16). A positive relationship has been shown between the trunk moment and the intragastric pressure, which tends to support this idea, but further studies of the exact relationship of intra-gastric pressure to disc compression is needed to analyze and test the hypothesis. Usually the pressure increase is brief when an activity is carried out. Therefore, a more sustained support to the spine can not be expected, at least not one of substantial magnitude.

Electromyographic studies

The numerous studies of trunk muscles using electromyography are limited by the difficulty of obtaining valid quantitative measures during movements. When standing, there is little activity in any of the trunk muscles. During forward flexion, the posterior back muscles are increasingly active as the trunk moment increases until full flexion is reached when they become electrically silent. In that position, therefore, the trunk moment is resisted passively by ligaments and stretched muscles. It has been suggested that this increases the risk of injury, although no complete clinical evidence exists. While the trunk muscles on both sides of the spine act together in flexion-extension movements, there is considerable asymmetry in lateral bending and rotation.

Occupational biomechanics

Occupational biomechanics is important because of the injury mechanisms believed to result in low back pain, and because of the close relationship between work and low back disability (Chaffin and Andersson, 1984; Pope et al., 1984). The purpose of this discussion is to review some basic biomechanical problems and consequences of work activities as they relate to the spine. We will discuss the spinal biomechanics of posture, manual handling, and vibration (repetitive loading), but we will first consider the possible injury mechanisms leading to low back pain in an occupational environment.

Mechanical injury mechanisms or the cause of low back injury

At least three injury models present themselves as possible causes of low back pain in industry: single overload, repetitive loading, and static loading. Single overloads can occur through direct trauma (extrinsic) or overexertion (intrinsic). Direct trauma is an uncommon cause of low back pain in industry. Overexertion on the other hand is a common cause according to statistical data. For example, in the United States official statistics indicate that overexertion is the cause in 60% of low back pain patients and that about 500,000 workers are injured by overexertion each year. These data, although impressive in magnitude, do not allow distinction between single overload injuries and repetitive load injuries. These are believed to be caused by fatigue failure. The risk of overexertion injuries is influenced by age, fatigue, and concomitant diseases and thus the load level at which injury occurs varies greatly. Fatigue failure is also influenced by rest/work relationships because incomplete injuries can heal without ever being noticed.

Static loading is believed to cause injury by interference with the blood circulation (nutrition) of muscle, ligament and disc tissue.

One of the problems in dealing with back "injuries" is the inability to objectively identify the injury both in location and magnitude. This has severe effects on the patient/physician relationship. The patient wants a specific diagnosis and the physician is unable to provide it. As discussed elsewhere, it is important to not overdramatize the injury, but to deal with it quickly and appropriately. Further, once the acute stages of "injury" are over activity will promote healing, not prevent it. Three occupational factors are particularly implicated as causes of low back pain in industry: posture, lifting, and vibration.

Posture

Posture should be considered in terms of the predominant work posture (sitting, standing or walking), in terms of acquired postures (bending and

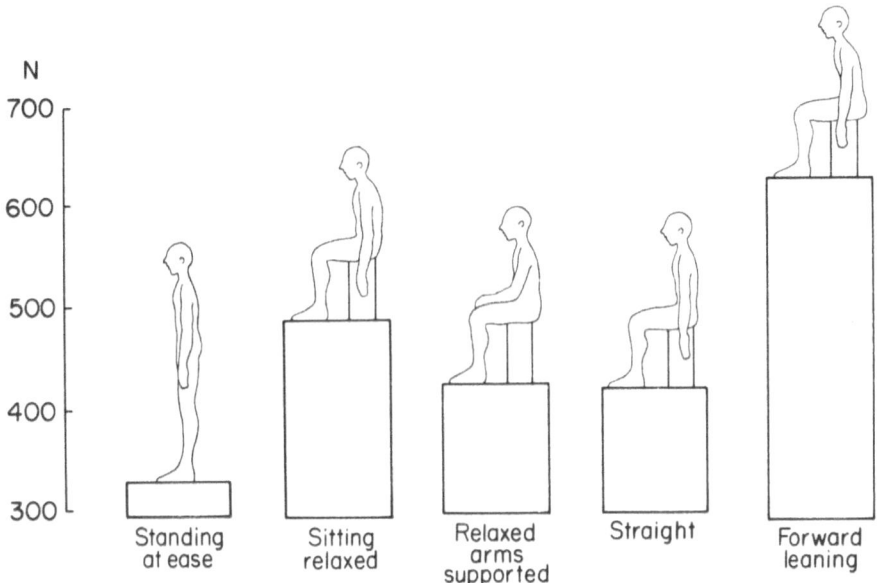

Fig. 17. Loads on the L 3 disc calculated from disc pressure measurements. (Adapted from Andersson et al., 1974)

twisting), and in terms of postural constraint. Biomechanical studies have shown that standing is less stressful to the spine than unsupported sitting (Fig. 17). This is because when sitting down the pelvis rotates backward and the spine flattens and deforms (Fig. 18). Sitting in well supported postures, however, with chairs providing back support, particularly for the lumbar region, is less stressful to the back than standing (Fig. 19). Flexion of the trunk results in high loads on the spine, increasing as the trunk moment increases. Twisting is also stressful not least because of the asymmetry in load occuring in asymmetric postures.

Postural constraints particularly from sitting in unchanged positions for long periods of time can cause postural fatigue and low back pain. This is particularly the case in the new computerized office setting where complaints of low back, neck and shoulder pain are quite frequent.

Lifting

Lifting is stressful to the spine because of the load moment. This means that not only the weight of the load should be considered, but also the location of that weight and the posture of the trunk. Thus, the two principle moments acting on the spine in lifting are: (1) the moment due to body segments (trunk, head, arms, hands) which can be estimated from the weight of these body

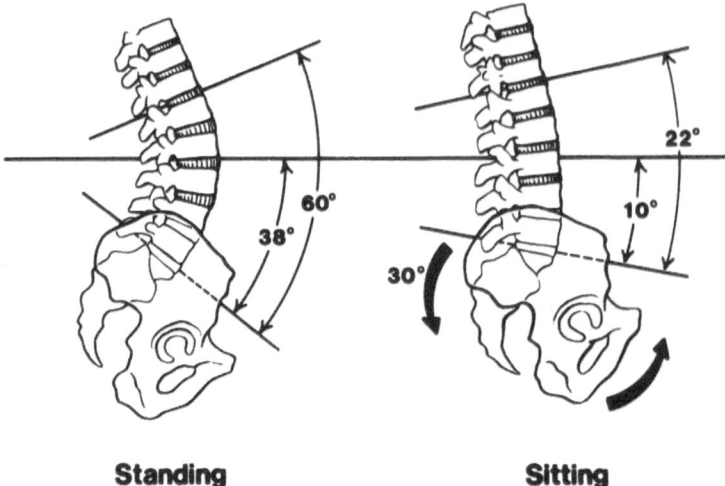

Fig. 18. When sitting down the pelvis rotates backwards and the lumbar spine flattens. (Adapted from Andersson et al., 1978)

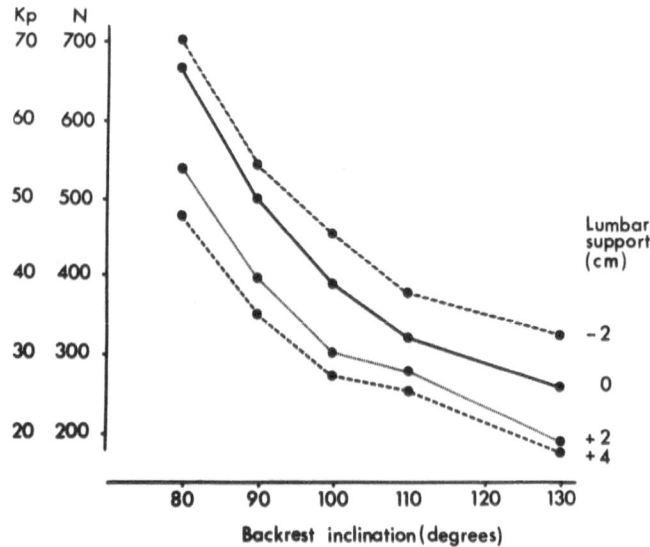

Fig. 19. An increase in backrest inclination, and in lumbar spine support results in a decrease in load on the L3 disc. Calculated from disc pressure measurements. (Adapted from Andersson et al., 1974)

segments and the moment arms from the spine to their centers of gravity, and (2) the moment due to the load, which is the product of the weight of the load and its moment arm (distance from load center of mass to spine). Because of the weight of the upper body the moment due to body posture usually far exceeds the moment due to the load. This means that the important factors to be controlled in lifting are (1) the posture which should be as upright as possible with the arms and hands as close to the body as possible, and (2) the location and weight of the external load which should be lifted close to the body. In many situations this can best be accomplished using a lifting technique called leg lifting where the knees are bent and the trunk upright. If the load cannot be brought in close to the body leg lifting will increase the load on the spine, however.

Other important factors in regard to lifting are the speed of the lift – the faster the lift the higher the load on the spine – and the symmetry of the lift – to avoid asymmetric loading of the spine.

Several factors influence a particular individual's capacity to lift. They include age, sex, lean body mass, conditioning, training, strength, and previous injuries. Thus, the safety of lifting (and pulling, pushing, and carrying) is not easy to generalize; there is no single value. Lifting aids should be used when possible, and the frequency of lifts should also be limited to avoid fatigue injuries. And, as often as possible lifting should be done by two persons.

Vibration

Vibration affects the spine by causing mechanical fatigue to spinal tissues, and perhaps also by interfering with nutrition. When the frequency of the vibration (for example in a car) is the same as the natural frequency of the spine (about 4.5–5 Hz) resonance occurs which increases the stresses on the spinal structures. Impulse loading from uneven surfaces can be sufficient to fracture vertebrae, particularly when osteoporosis is present.

Pathology of intervertebral discs and apophyseal joints (facet joints)

Several changes take place in the discs and facet joints with age. They are to be viewed as normal aging but can have negative consequences for the adjacent tissues, and can result in pain. The composition of the disc is similar to other cartilage tissue. It consists of sparsely distributed cells in a matrix of collagen and proteoglycans. The disc changes its morphology and chemical composition with time. Thus there is a gradual reduction in water content from 80% at birth in the annulus and 90% in the nucleus to 70 and 75% respectively by the third decade. From this time on the annulus retains its water content, while the nucleus continues to progressively lose water till its content approaches that of the annulus.

At birth the nucleus comprises most of the disc. It is gelatinous and bulges spontaneously from a cut surface. Only 15% of its dry weight is collagen. By the third decade, however, most of its gelatinous appearance is lost and the nucleus is invaded by collagen from the inner layers of the annulus. Progressively, a loss in proteoglycan content occurs leading to a change in the collagen to proteoglycan relationship. After middle age, splits and clefts can often be seen in the disc. They are usually, at first, oriented parallel to the endplates and are found in the center of the disc. These clefts increase with time and can lead to an isolation of a central part of a disc which then appears almost as a loose body (Vernon-Roberts, 1978). The clefts usually extend more dorsally than anteriorly and sometimes extend to the posterior annulus, occasionally penetrating all annular layers. Vernon-Roberts, when dissecting discs post-mortem, also found circumferential tears in the posterolateral areas of the annulus. Another frequent finding were the so called Schmorl's nodes believed to be herniations of disc material into the vertebral bodies (Fig. 20). In the spines examined by Vernon-Roberts and Pirie (1977) Schmorl's nodes were present in 50%, and a posterior prolapse in 10%. While Schmorl's nodes were often present without degeneration of the disc, herniations were usually associated with degenerative changes. These herniations seem to occur when the disc is still semi-gelatinous and are rare when desiccation and collagenization of the nucleus has occurred.

As we age and the disc loses its water, it also loses height. Osteophytes (bony projections) also occur with increasing age as part of the degenerative process (Fig. 21). These osteophytes are most frequently found at the anterolateral border of the vertebral bodies and generally increase in size with increasing severity of the degenerative process. Posterior osteophytes are less common, but can compromise the lateral intervertebral foraminae when located posterolaterally (Chap. 9).

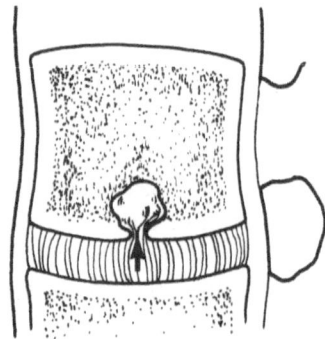

Fig. 20. Illustration of a Schmorl's node

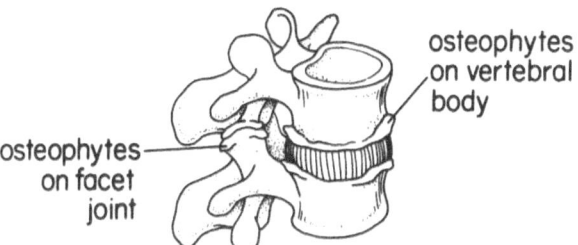

Fig. 21. With degeneration osteophytes occur both at the vertebra-disc junctions and at the facet joints. (Adapted from Fine, 1985)

Severe degenerative changes in the disc are often accompanied by osteoarthritic changes in the apophyseal joints (facet joints). On the other hand, degenerative changes in these joints rarely, if ever, occur when the disc is not degenerated. This suggests that the osteoarthritic process is usually secondary, and probably the result of a change in stress distribution. As degeneration progresses, cartilage degrades in the facet joints and osteophytes develop which not infrequently grow into the intervertebral foraminae creating a situation of spinal stenosis.

The role of the disc in the pathogensis of low back pain

The assumption that most episodes of acute low back pain are discogenic in origin is supported by circumstantial evidence, pathologic studies, biomechanical studies, experimental studies, and some direct in vivo observations. The clinical (circumstantial) evidence that the disc is a frequent source of lower back pain stems from the observation that patients who experience acute disc herniations frequently give the history of having had one or more acute episodes of lower back pain prior to the herniation. The first episode of low back pain may have been many years previously, however, and may have been forgotten. Nonetheless, many patients vividly recall the initial episode, its cause, and duration. They also frequently will have experienced multiple recurrences of varying intensity. Adding to this circumstantial evidence is the fact that patients who have experienced multiple episodes of lower back pain often have been followed for many years including multiple X-rays. Radiologic changes in the disc will then eventually become evident. Although this could well have happened without back pain the conclusion is often made that the pain is based on these changes. It is quite clear, however, that degenerative changes do not have to result in back pain. Indeed they are as frequent in patients without as in patients with back pain. Structurally, chemically and biomechanically, we cannot distinguish between a disc which has degenerated and is pain-free and one that is symptom producing.

In vivo experiments have convincingly demonstrated that typical lumbar pain and sciatica can be produced by manipulations of the annulus or the nerve root, and by injections into the disc. Nerve endings can be found in all of the structures of the lumbar spine except in the nucleus pulposis. Painful manipulation of the ligamentous and bony structures of the lumbar spine produces a characteristic pattern of referral to the region of the sacroiliac joints, buttock, groin, and upper thigh. Typical sciatica is only produced by stimulation of the annulus or nerve root (Hirsch et al., 1963). This does not preclude the possibility that stimulation of these structures, without disc prolapse, might produce other typical lumbar pain syndromes.

Figure 22 demonstrates the relationship between low back pain, annular tear, and the later development of radiologic evidence of degenerative changes. The later development of radiologic changes is typical of every joint in which there has been significant cartilage injury and is not typical of only the lumbar spine.

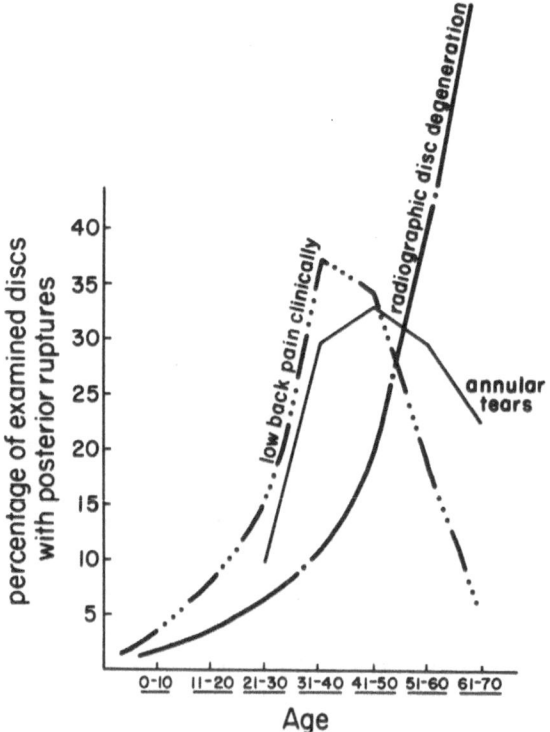

Fig. 22. The frequency of annular tears in the lumbar region compared to radiographic disc degeneration and low back pain as a function of age. (Adapted from Hirsch and Schajowicz, 1952)

Pain

The study of the initiation, transmission, and the preception of pain has been advanced to a remarkable degree through the study of the neural receptors and the chemical mediators that are responsible for the conduction of an impulse from one nerve cell to another; and, conversely, the inhibition of this transmission. A great impetus to our understanding of pain has come from the study of opiate receptors in the central nervous system (Snyder et al., 1986); and, to a lesser extent, the study of bradykinin and prostaglandins peripherally.

Highly specific localization of mechanical impulses originate in the periphery in mechanoreceptors and are transmitted via rapidly conducting (A-delta) myelinated fibers with few synapses to the thalamus and then to the cerebral cortex (Fig. 23). These are a component of the "new" (neospinalthalamic) portion of the nervous system and are conducted to the ventral posterio-lateral (VPL) nucleus of the thalamus with few synapses. In the VPL nucleus the neurones are organized in a manner designed to localize the source of the input from the periphery. Interaction between the VPL nucleus and the posterior and medial thalamus localizes the source of the painful input. The pain perception that arises from the stimulus of the A-delta fibers is rapid in onset, "bright" in character, and of relatively short duration (Chapman and Bonica, 1983) (Table 3).

Simultaneous stimulation of other large, rapidly conducting, myelinated fibers (mechanoreceptors) may modulate the input from smaller nociceptors.

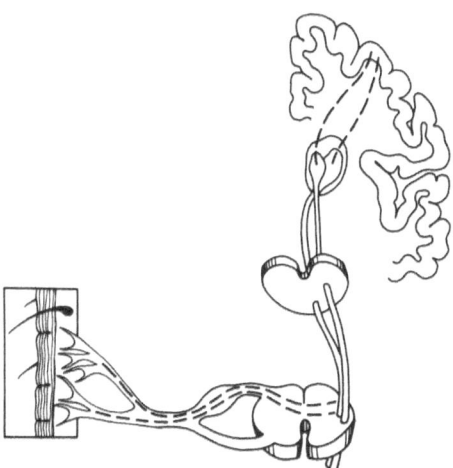

Fig. 23. Pain path in the rapidly conducting system. Pain arises in the periphery from mechanoreceptors and is transmitted via myelinated fibers to the thalamus and cerebral cortex

Table 3. Difference between pain arising from the rapidly conducting fibers (fast pain) and the slowly conducting fibers (slow pain)

Fast pain	Slow pain
Well localized	Poorly localized
Short duration	Long duration
Sharp	Dull
Little emotion	Emotional response
Short latency	Longer latency
Not blocked by morphine	Blocked by morphine
Neospinothalamic system	Paleospinothalamic system

At the "gate" in the substantia gelatinosa of the posterior horn of the spinal cord the impulse from the myelinated fibers may inhibit the transmission from the small nociceptor fibers (Fig. 24). Inhibition of the small fiber transmission also may take place via exogenous opiates and via powerful central inhibition through descending corticospinal tracts (Fig. 25). The opiates act directly upon receptors in the substantia gelatinosa (and centrally) while the descending tracts provide analgesic function in response to information processed in the higher centers. The rapidly conducting large myeli-

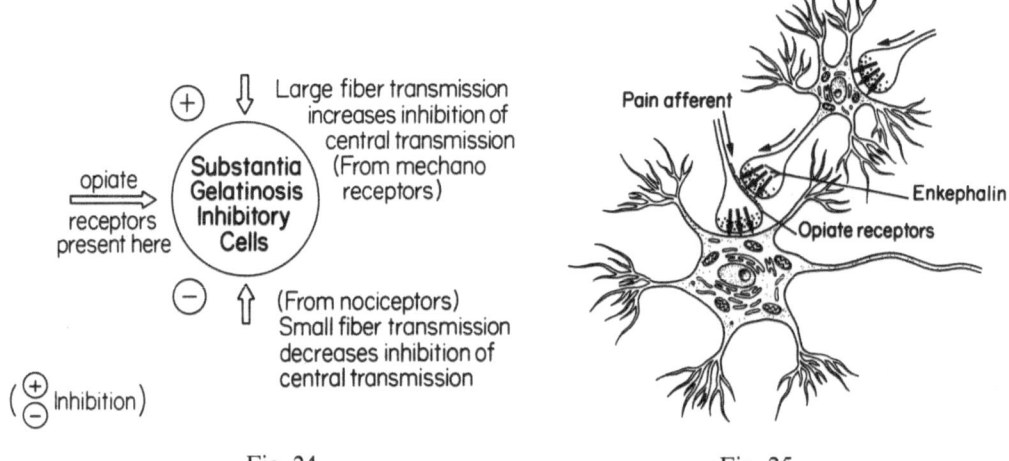

Fig. 24   Fig. 25

Fig. 24. Gate control theory of pain

Fig. 25. Pain transmission can be inhibited by opiates acting on receptors in the substantia gelatinosa and centrally. (Adapted form Snyder et al., 1985)

nated fibers bring information transmitted via the small fibers. Inhibition of the painful impulse is therefore possible before conscious perception of the nociceptor impulse. Conversely, central (cord) mechanisms may exist which allow persistent pain impulses to be conducted via the spinal cord in the absence of impulses from the periphery as in the case of "phantom limb", or deafferentation as in dorsal rizotomy.

In 1965, Melzak and Wall presented the "Gate control theory" of pain transmission (Fig. 24). This theory has undergone modification since that time, but the basic concept has continued to provide a useful tool for the understanding of the transmission of the painful impulse and its modification and inhibition. It has become evident that the theory does not present a complete picture of pain transmisssion or perception as it leaves out modulating mechanisms which are present peripheral to the dorsal horn and also lacks necessary emphasis on the important central modulating mechanisms (Engel, 1983; Maciewicz and Sandrew, 1985). For the purposes of this book a rather general explanation of the mechanism of pain impulse transmission, modulation and inhibition will be used.

In the periphery the free nerve endings have a high threshold and a significant delay before transmission begins. These nerve endings are called nociceptors since they signal imminent tissue injury. The impulse may be initiated by tissue humoral factors including bradykinin and prostaglandins (Snyder et al., 1986). The impulse is conducted via small fibers (C-unmyelinated) which are part of the "old" (paleospinal-thalamic) portion of the nervous system (Table 3). These free endings are sensitive to all types of stimulation (e.g., pressure, temperature). Many synaptic relays are interposed between the free nerve ending and the eventual reception by the cerebral cortex. Each free nerve ending has several synaptic junctions in the substantia gelatinosa in the dorsal horn of the spinal cord. From there connection is made with the ascending spinothalamic tract of the cord. These fibers may terminate in the nuclei of the brain stem, in the periaqueductal grey matter, or in the posterior or media thalmus. The impulses arriving via this portion (paleospinothalamic system) are not coded as to the source of the input. The pain input via this system is slow in onset, dull in character, and persistent. Both inhibition and accentuation appear to take place under certain circumstances.

Opiate receptors have been discovered in the substance gelatinosa of the spinal cord, the media thalmus, the periaqueductal grey matter, and the limbic system. It was then postulated that there must be opiate-like neurotransmittors naturally occurring in the central nervous system which would have an affinity for these receptors. Even before their discovery these neurotransmitters were given the name "endorphines" meaning "internal morphines". Several different polypeptides have been discovered which bind to the opiate receptors in the central nervous system. These have the effect of blocking a portion of the pain impulse at the level of the spinal cord, but they also have a much wider effect in the brain as a central mediator of pain response and a variety of emotional responses. It is wider limbic system connection to the pain response and the opiate receptor system which appears to hold the explanation for the addictive nature of opiate-like drugs and possibly some aspects of the phenomena of chronic pain behavior.

The low back syndromes and their interpretation

The symptom of pain in the lower back is most often related to the structures of the lumbar spine, sacrum, and their associated muscular and nervous structures. However, there are many other structures which, when they become diseased, may refer pain to the lower back. Examples are dissection of an abdominal aortic aneurysm, posterior penetration of a duodenal ulcer, renal calculus, and endometriosis. Less common examples are retroperitoneal fibrosis, lymphoma, and malignant diseases of the pelvis. This book attempts to divide the general symptom of "low back pain" into recognizable syndromes in order to provide the clinical physician with a tool for rapid and accurate judgment when confronted with this complaint. It is commonly stated that less than ten percent of back pains ever have a diagnosis other than a description of the presenting syndrome. We believe that it is reasonable and proper to relate a given syndrome to the most probable underlying pathology even though scientific proof does not always exist. This is the only way in which the physician can render reasonable treatment, offer a prognosis, and teach prevention. The common medical attitude is that if there is not a systemic disease causing the back ache then the cause of the symptom will probably remain indeterminate. It is just this vagueness that results in prolonged treatment, iatrogenic disability, and unnecessary surgical remedies.

2 Investigations

In collaboration with G. D. Dobben

Patient history and physical examination

Patient history

The patient's description of his or her problem is the key to the evaluation. In this text, specific low back syndromes are discussed in individual chapters. Differentiating between them requires a careful patient interview. Specifics to look for in individual patients are discussed in the chapters below. The subsequent discussion is generic to the obtainment of a history in any low back patient.

The sequence of the interview is not essential, but logically starts with the present problem (the reason for the patient's visit) and then proceeds to discuss previous lower back problems, the patient's general medical condition, and previous medical and surgical problems. A short socioeconomic and work related history should also be obtained.

A detailed description of the patient's present problem should include how it started, what was initially done, and how it did progress. Patients tend to describe some trauma related to the onset but this is not necessarily the cause of the patient's back problem. For legal reasons the circumstances and severity of work and traffic accident related pain should always be documented carefully.

As with any painful condition, the most important information is related to the patient's pain. Pain intensity, location (distribution), and pattern are important variables as is information about activities that increase or decrease pain. The severity can be expressed verbally or recorded on a visual analog scale (Fig. 1). Pain location and radiation can be described or illustrated on a pain drawing (Fig. 2). The intensity of pain, changes of pain over the day, and reaction to activities are important clues to diagnosis. Most back

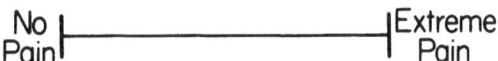

Fig. 1. A visual-analog scale used to record pain. The patient crosses off at a point on the line corresponding to the intensity of pain

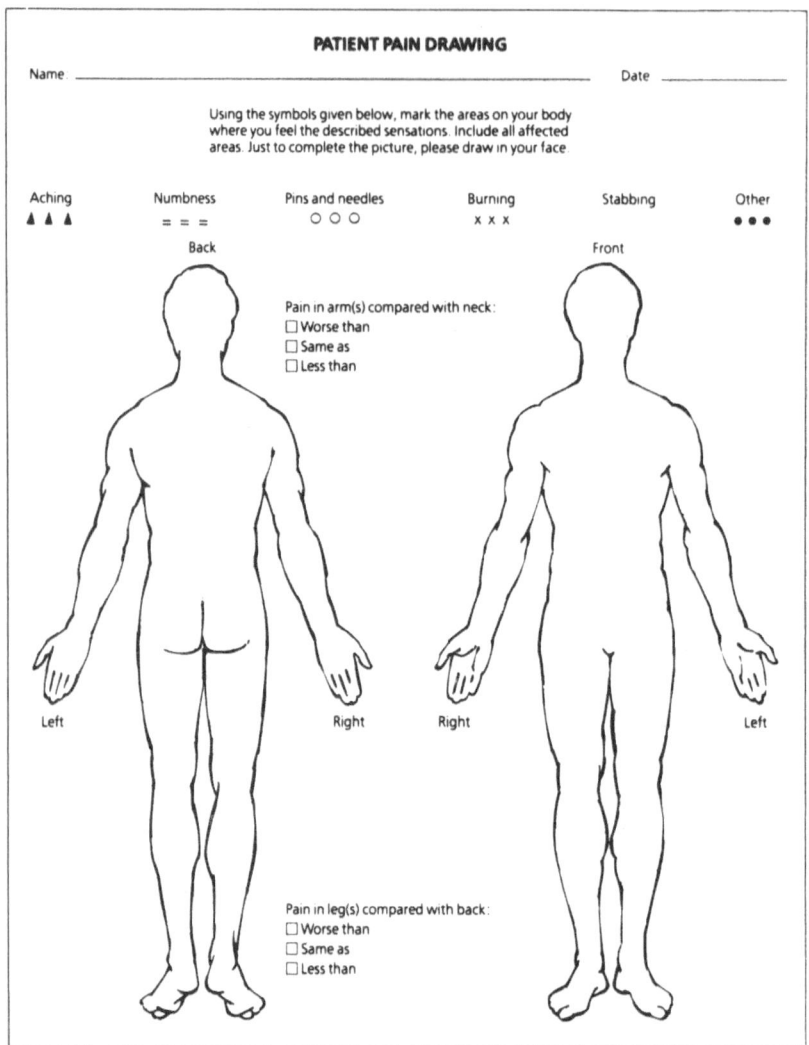

Fig. 2. An example of a pain drawing. The patient fills in the symbols at the appropriate areas. (Adapted from the Univ. of Texas, Southwestern Medical School, Orthopaedic Division, Spine Care Program)

conditions improve with rest and deteriorate with activity. For further discussion see the individual syndrome chapters. The quality of pain is also important as is information about parasthesias (pins and needles) and numbness. Bowel and bladder dysfunctions are extremely important considerations (see Chap. 8). Previous back problems, surgeries, treatments and response to those should also be reviewed.

The patient's general condition is also important. Are there other reasons than spinal to the patient's pain? Is there a reason to suspect metastatic or other malignant disease? Are there infectious processes anywhere in the body? Does the patient present with fever, chills, and weight loss? Is the patient's problem due to a general metabolic disease? Does the patient take medications? All of these are questions that should be considered.

Since socioeconomic factors are important in back conditions, some information should be obtained. Life stress factors may aggravate disease. Disability benefits and litigation can negatively influence recovery.

The patient's work and education also need to be reviewed. Is it realistic to return the patient to his previous job after recovery? Is, in fact, the patient's back problem triggered by work-related factors?

During the interview, observations of the patient can give important clues. Discomfort, pain behaviour, depression, and signs of alcohol abuse are such clues that are useful to the evaluation and treatment.

In patients with psychological factors further specific tests may be required. These are discussed in Chap. 13.

Physical examination

The physical examination of the lumbar spine and the lower extremities in patients with low back pain and/or sciatica is fundamental to diagnostic and treatment decisions. The examination described below should be viewed as a minimum examination which in specific cases and for the application of specific treatment need to be supplemented by additional tests.

The examination can conveniently follow the routine described in Table 1, starting with the patient standing and then moving on to examining the patient sitting and finally lying down first on the back and then on the abdomen. The examination involves inspection, palpation, determination of range of motion, and a few neurologic tests.

Inspection

The patient should be barefoot at the time of examination and dressed such that the entire length of the spine can be observed. Inspection should include observation of the patient's gait, including the ability to stand on toes and heels. The surface of the back is observed for pigmented spots (cafe au lait), localized blisters (herpes zoster), and other abnormalities. The posture is then inspected not only from the back, but also from the sides and the front. The following should be recorded:

(1) The position of the head in the frontal and sagittal planes.

(2) The level of the scapula and shoulders in the frontal plane.

(3) The configuration of the spine in terms of lordosis, kyphosis, and scoliosis (Fig. 3). The presence of a list is also recorded.

Table 1. Physical examination of the spine. Organization of a routine

Patient standing	inspection
	palpation
	range of motion
	gait (toe and heel)
Patient sitting	straight leg raising
	patella reflexes
	achilles reflexes
	quadriceps strength
Patient lying supine	straight leg raising
	Lasegue's test
	hip ROM
	lower extremity reflexes
	motor function
	sensory function
	Babinski test
	leg length
	circumference
	abdominal examination
	peripheral pulses
Patient lying prone	palpation
	SI joint stress test

(4) The level of the iliac crest in the sagittal plane and in the transverse plane. If there is a difference between the right and the left side frontal plane, this should be corrected by placing appropriate size-blocks under the shortened extremity and the leg length difference should be recorded.

(5) Muscle hypotrophies and obvious areas of muscle contractions.

(6) The configuration of the lower extremities including varus and vagus deformities of the knees and ankle, flexion-extension deformities of the knee and hip joints and internal and external rotation of the hip joints.

Palpation

Palpation of the spine is done to detect muscle spasms which would tend to make the paravertebral muscles extraordinarily firm and sometimes bulging. Local masses should also be palpated for. Local tenderness should be determined by palpation over the spinous processes, the muscles, and over the iliac crests and sacrum. Tenderness at the sciatic notch is also determined.

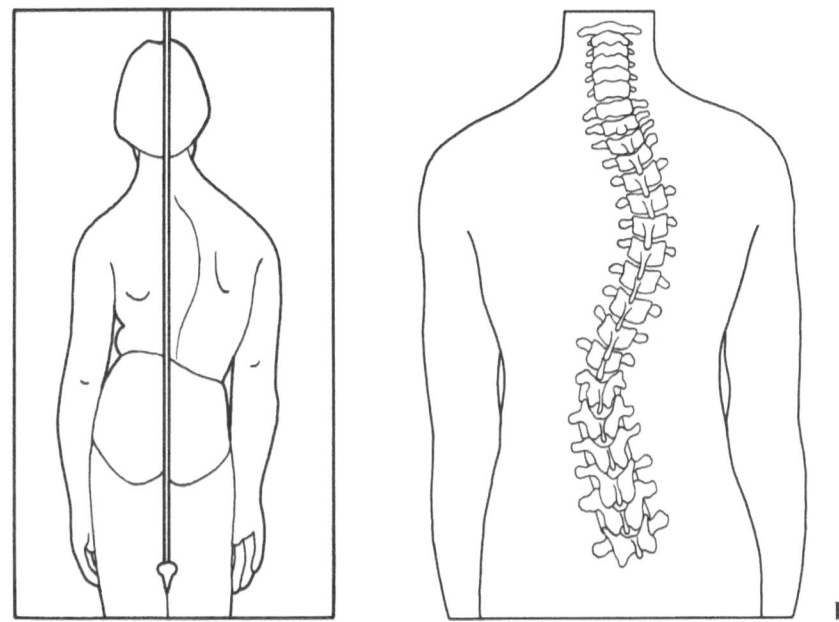

Fig. 3. a Patient with scoliosis. A plump-bob can be used to measure deviation.
b Vertebral body configuration in a patient with scoliosis

Range of motion (ROM)

Range of motion is determined with the patient standing and the examiner observing from the back. During the examination, the pattern of motion is also recorded and the patient is told to express whether or not pain occurs. We suggest starting the examination with the patient bending forward and backward. This motion should first be done with the examiner just viewing the flexion-extension movement and then during simultaneous palpation which makes it easier to detect any olisthesis. The examination is then continued with lateral bending and finally rotation. To isolate rotation to the lumbar spine, the pelvis should be stabilized either by the examiner's hands holding the iliac crests or by determining rotation with the patient sitting. Determination of the precise range of motion of the lumbar spine is difficult and has led to the development of several different methods. It appears that at the present time the use of either the pendulum goniometer or a flexible ruler provides the most reliable and repeatable measure (Fig. 4). Measurement of changes in the length of the lumbar spine also frequently used (Fig. 5) but involves problems particularly in obese patients and also does not allow for measurements of lateral flexion and rotation. Since forward flexion is a combined movement of the spine and pelvis, measurements of the distance to the floor are not accurate in determining the range of movement of the

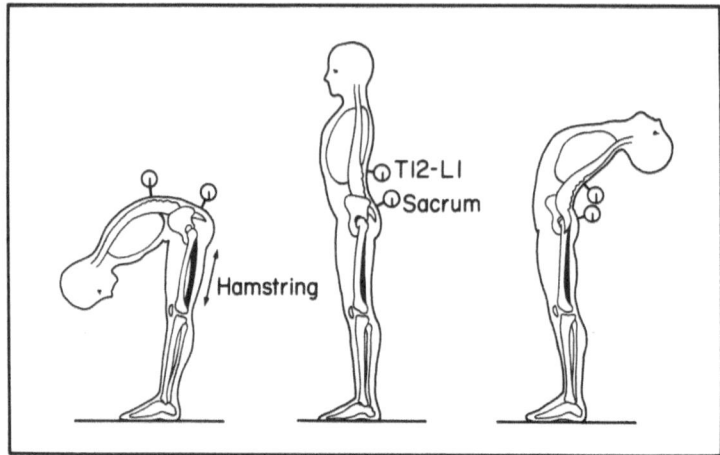

Fig. 4. Range of motion measured with two goniometers. Since flexion and extension are combined, movements of hip joints and spine both must be measured to determine true spine motion, and then the hip motion (*sacrum*) be subtracted from the total motion (*T12-L1*). (Adapted from Mayer, 1985)

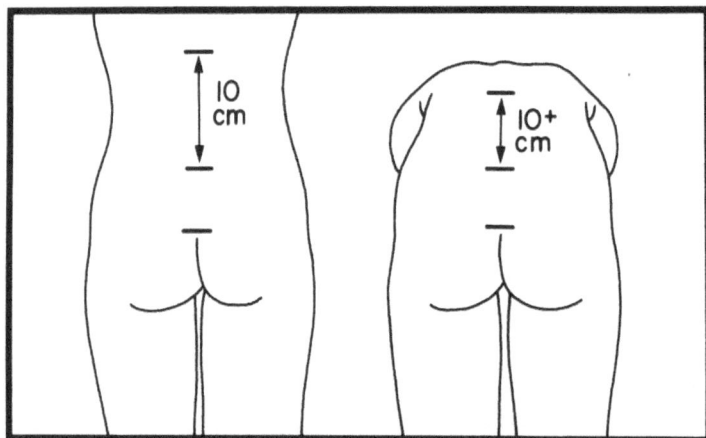

Fig. 5. Range of motion measured as a change in distance between sacrum and a lumbar vertebra

lumbar spine. Further, to determine the true flexion-extension movement of the spine, trunk and pelvic movements will have to be determined and then pelvic movement subtracted from trunk movement (Fig. 4). Lateral bending is sometimes observed by having the patient move the hand down along the length of the leg and then measuring the distance to the floor (Fig. 6). Asymmetries may be important indicators of the location, e.g., of a disc herniation.

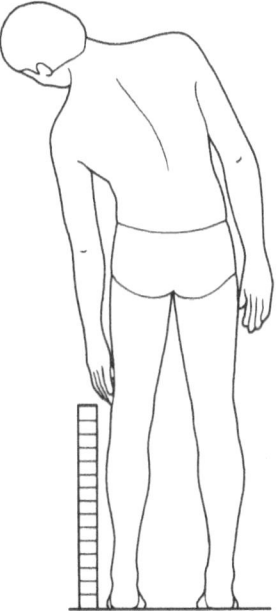

Fig. 6. Lateral bending

Straight leg raising (SLR)

With a patient sitting, SLR is tested as well as patellar and achilles reflexes. The sitting straight leg raise test involves extending the leg with the patient sitting on the examination couch. The patient is then asked to lie down on the back. In this position, the straight leg raise is repeated lifting one leg at a time from the examination table and recording the angle at which pain occurs. The knee should be extended and it should be recorded whether pain occurs in the lower back or in the leg (Fig. 7). To increase the stretch of the sciatic nerve, extension of the ankle joint can be performed at the same time. A positive straight leg raise test should be distinguished from inability to extend the leg due to hamstring muscle tightness. Raising of the unaffected leg in patients with sciatica can sometimes cause pain in the opposite leg. This is called a positive contralateral straight leg raise test. Lasegue's sign is another test performed to test for sciatic nerve involvement. In this test, the hip and knee are both flexed 90°. From that position, the knee joint is extended recording the degree of extension at which pain occurs. Hip joint range of motion can conveniently be determined subsequent to the straight leg raise test. Since pain arising from the hip joints is sometimes quite similar to pain arising from the lower back in its distribution, hip ROM is an important test not to be omitted.

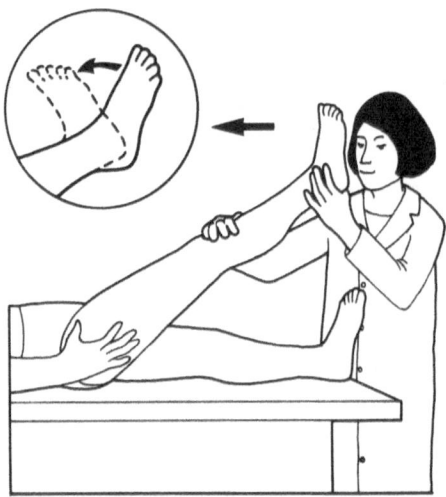

Fig. 7. Straight leg raising test

Neurologic examination

The neurologic examination in patients with back pain and sciatica involves testing for lower leg reflexes, motor function, and sensation. Most lower back disorders causing neurologic changes in the lower extremities either influence the patella and achilles reflexes or the strength of the extensor hallucis longus. Neurologic changes associated with common lumbar disc herniations are recorded in Table 2 and also appear in Figs. 8, 9, and 10.

The patellar or quadriceps reflex is elicited when the patellar tendon is firmly tapped. It is the response of the quadriceps femoris muscle and requires an intact L4 spinal nerve. The achilles or triceps surae reflex, also termed the ankle jerk, is elicited by firmly tapping the achilles tendon. An absence of this reflex indicates an S1 nerve root involvement. The triceps surae reflex can also be elicited by tapping under the plantar aspect of the foot, the so-called plantar reflex. Sometimes the tibialis posterior reflex is also elicited. This is done by tapping the tibialis posterior tendon behind the medial malleolus and results in an inversion of the foot. It is primarily a test of the L5 nerve root. Brisk or weak reflexes should not be interpreted as abnormal, particularly if the reflexes are symmetrical. Sometimes the reflex has to be reinforced by the so-called Jendrassik's maneuver in which the patient hooks the fingers of both hands together pulling the fingers apart as the tendon is tapped.

The most important motor function to determine is the extension power of the extensor hallucis longus. A reduction in extension power indicates involvement of the L5 nerve root. The test is done by asking the patient to

Table 2. Lumbar radicular syndrome

Disc level:	Any central disc herniation	L5/S1	L4/5	L3/4
Nerve root involved:	cauda equina (L4/5 > L5/S1)	S1	L5	L4
Pain referral pattern:	perineum low back buttocks either or both legs	unilateral low back buttocks posterior leg	unilateral low back buttocks lateral leg and tigh	unilateral low back buttocks posterolateral leg
Motor deficit:	unilateral or bilateral leg weakness	unilateral weakness plantar flexion of foot; difficulty with toe walking	unilateral weakness dorsiflexion of foot; difficulty with heel walking	unilateral quadriceps weakness
Sensory deficit:	perineum/ buttocks low back thighs, legs, feet	lateral foot, postero-lateral calf	lateral calf; between 1st and 2nd toe	knee distal anterior thigh
Reflexes compromised:	ankle jerk	ankle jerk	0	knee jerk

extend the big toe and hold firmly while pulling down on both toes at the same time. The extensor digitorum muscles (also innervated by L5) can be tested at the same time by pulling the whole foot downward. Plantar flexion strength, the loss of which would indicate an S1 root involvement, and inversion-eversion strength can also be tested. The loss of eversion strength would primarily indicate that an S1 nerve root involvement, while the loss of inversion strength would indicate an L4 root involvement. Quadriceps strength is determined by having the patient extend the lower leg against resistance.

The neurologic examination should also include the Babinski test which is elicited by stimulating the plantar skin of the foot from the heel forward (Fig. 11). When the toes flex, the response is negative. If the big toe extends, however, the test is positive, indicating an upper motor neuron lesion.

The sensation of the lower legs is tested to determine whether specific dermatomes are affected or not (Fig. 12). As discussed subsequently, a sensory pattern which does not correspond to the anatomic nerve distribution is an important observation.

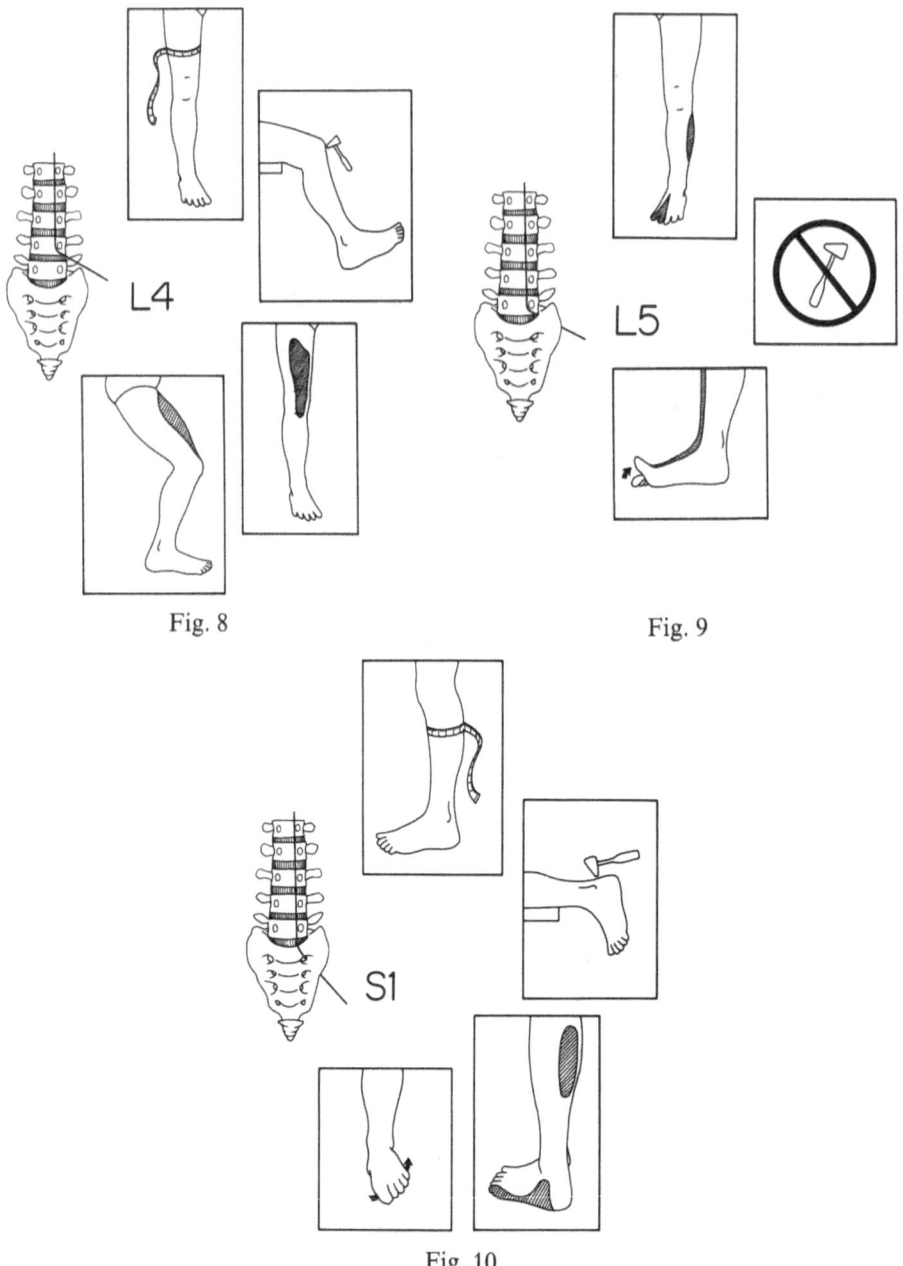

Fig. 8

Fig. 9

Fig. 10

Fig. 8. The L4 syndrome is characterized by loss of the quadriceps reflex and some-times weakness and atrophy of the quadriceps muscle. Typical sensory changes are also illustrated

Fig. 9. The L5 syndrome is characterized by weakness in the extensor hallucis longus (and sometimes the extensor digitorum). The lower extremity reflexes are normal. Typical sensory changes are also illustrated

Fig. 10. The S1 syndrome is characterized by absence of the ankle reflex, and some-times eversion strength. Typical sensory changes are also illustrated

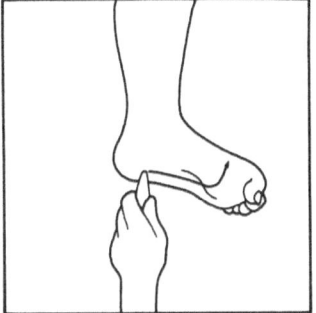 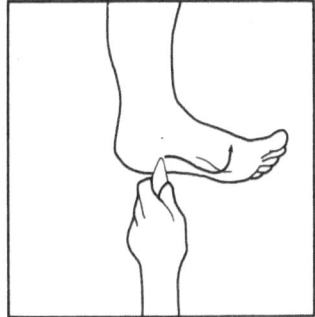

Fig. 11. Babinski's test. (Positive when the toes extend)

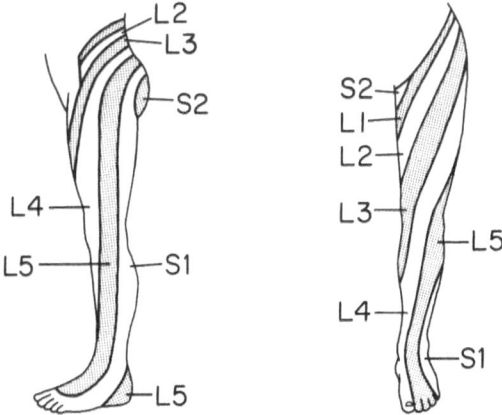

Fig. 12. Sensory dermatomes

Atrophies are rare. To detect early atrophies measurements of circumferences at specific distances below and above the knee joints must be obtained.

In our opinion, most patients can be evaluated with an abbreviated neurologic exam involving eliciting the patellar and achilles reflexes, determining the motor function of the extensor hallucis longus and the sensory functions of the lower extremities.

Sacroiliac joint tests

With a patient prone on the examination table, the spinal processes are again palpated noting tenderness, or any other abnormality. Further, the sacroiliac joints and the buttocks areas are also palpated noting tenderness and abnormal masses. The sacroiliac joints can be tested in the prone position by placing the fingers of one hand on one side of the pelvis and using the other

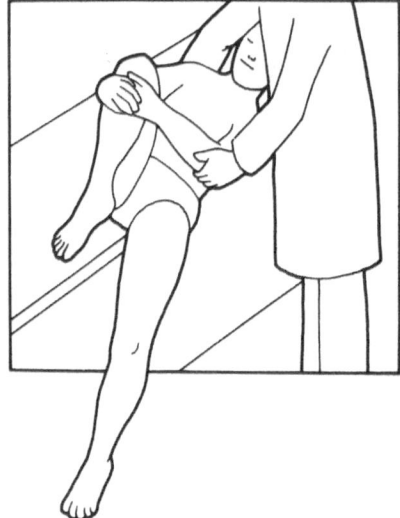

Fig. 13. Gaenslen's test

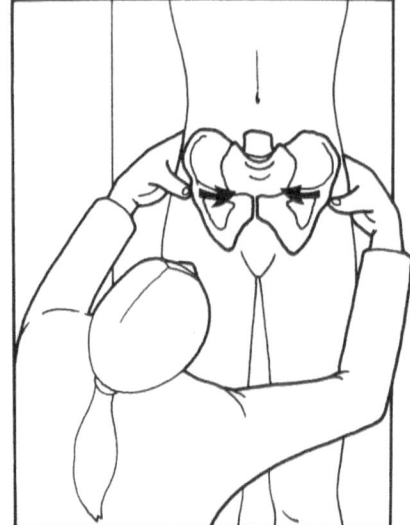

Fig. 14. Pelvic rock test

hand to raise opposite leg. Other tests to specifically stress the sacroiliac joints include the Gaenslen test, which is performed with the patient recumbent and involves hyperextending one leg while the pelvis and lumbar spine are fixed by means of extreme flexion of the opposite leg (Fig. 13). If pain occurs, the sacroiliac joints would be more likely to be the origin than the lumbosacral area. Pelvic rock tests (Fig. 14) can also be performed by compressing the pelvis at the superior iliac spine. Although numerous tests have been devised to test the sacroiliac joints, none is entirely specific.

Non-organic physical signs

A set of inappropriate responses to the examination referred to as non-organic physical signs has been proposed by Waddell et al. (1980). They are useful to determine malingering or exaggeration on the part of the patient. Tests of inappropriate response to the examination include:

(1) tenderness – superficial and nonanatomical;
(2) simulation – axial loading and simulated rotation;
(3) distraction – straight leg raising;
(4) regional – weakness and sensory disturbance;
(5) overreaction to examination.

Non-organic tenderness can express itself as extreme superficial tenderness to light pinching over a wide area of the lumbar spine or as deep tenderness over a wide area not localized to one structure. The simulation tests include axial loading in which the examiner is pushing down on the patient's skull or shoulders. This should not respond in significant lumbar pain (because the lower back is only mildly stressed), while pain in the neck may occur. Simulated rotation of the lumbar spine involves rotating the shoulder and pelvis together. When this is done rotation occurs in the hip joints. In the presence of nerve irritation, simulated rotation can cause leg pain but otherwise pain should not increase due to this motion. The distraction tests include straight leg raising, done sitting and standing or repeated SLR while distracting the patient in different ways. Regional disturbances such as giving way of many muscle groups, which cannot be explained on a neurological basis or sensory disturbances in a stocking pattern involving several nerve roots are other nonorganic signs. Over-reaction during the examination may take different forms, such as verbalization, facial expression, tremor, collapsing and sweating. Cultural differences can result in variations in these over-reactions. The inappropriate physical signs combined with other types of psychological tests are useful in differentiating between physical disease and magnified illness behaviour.

Other examinations

Chest expansion should be measured if ankylosing spondylitis is suspected. An expansion of less than 2.5 cm (1″) during inspiration is abnormal.

Abdominal palpation should be done to detect abdominal masses or tenderness.

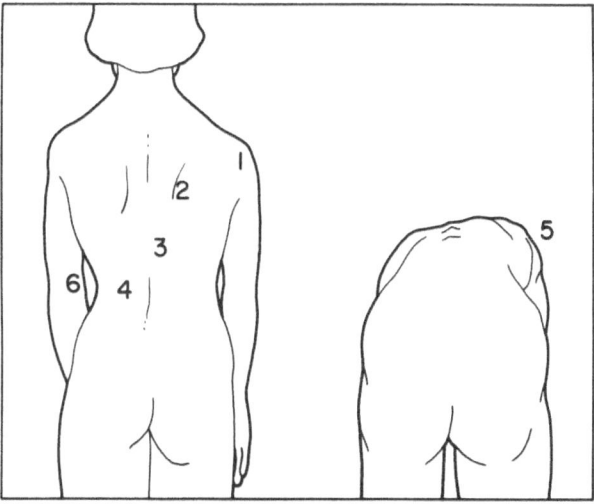

Fig. 15. Scoliosis checklist: *1* shoulder level, *2* scapular symmetry, *3* spinous process alignment, *4* flank symmetry, *5* thoracic symmetry, *6* evenness of hang of arms. (Adapted from Kane, 1977)

In patients with scoliosis a specific examination routine should be used as illustrated in Fig. 15.

Electrophysiologic tests

Electrodiagnostic tests include electromyography (EMG), nerve conduction studies and somatosensory evoked potentials (SEP). EMG and nerve conduction studies are sometimes used in patients with suspected nerve root compression syndromes. The values of such tests is uncertain, both because of low sensitivity and specificity. The addition of H reflexes and F responses have increased the value of electrodiagnostic studies. The H reflex is a response of the gastrocnemicus and soleus muscles to a submaximal stimulation of their motor nerve. The H reflex, like the Achilles tendon reflex, can be altered by nerve root lesions. At supramaximal levels of stimulation, the H reflex is inhibited and instead an F response generally appears. While electrodiagnostic tests have some value in diagnosis, they have generally been replaced by other tests such as myelography, CT scans, and MRIs. Many therefore feel that these tests are redundant. They can be helpful, however, in patients in whom sciatica persists and the structural diagnosis is uncertain. They can also be helpful in patients with metabolic disorders where the patients radiculopathy could be caused by their metabolic condition. Other patients in whom electrodiagnostics may be helpful are those in whom it is uncertain whether bladder dysfunction is caused by a spinal abnormality or not.

Because previous surgery influences the electrodiagnostic tests, and particularly electromyography, they are more difficult to interpret in patients who have undergone previous surgery.

SEPs are by some believed to have value in the diagnosis of spinal stenosis and in determining whether decompression in these patients has been adequate or not. The use of SEP as a diagnostic test remains controversial. Undoubtedly, they have some use in monitoring spinal cord function during operations in which spinal deformities are reduced and instrumented.

Thermography

Thermography is a method sometimes used to study patients with back pain. It is an appealing method since it is painless, non-invasive and without known adverse biological effects. Unfortunately scientific information to determine diagnostic reliability and validity is missing. The use of the method is highly controversial and, in our opinion, there is no indication for its use except in research, attempting to find out its true value.

Laboratory tests

Few laboratory tests are useful in patients with low back pain. Obviously, if metabolic disorders are considered, such tests are necessary and should be done (Chap. 17). However, in the average back patient, no laboratory tests are needed; although erythrocyte sedimentation rate (ESR) can be useful in screening patients in which the infections or tumors are suspected. The HLA-B27 histocompatibility antigen is present in 95% of patients with ankylosing spondylitis, and in a significant number of patients with other types of sero-negative inflammatory diseases (Chap. 17). HLA-B27 is not a useful screening test for patients with back pain and should only be ordered when clinical and radiographic suspicion exists.

Scintigraphy (isotope scans)

Scintigraphy is capable of providing morphological and metabolic information with very little risk to the patient. It is valuable in determining the presence or absence of osteomyelitis, metastatic and primary bone tumors, trauma, arthritis, metabolic bone diseases and discitis. Because bone scans can be done of the whole body at the same time, it is a convenient screening tool from which information can be obtained allowing more specific diagnostic tests to be made in the appropriate areas.

The bone seeking isotopes used in scintigraphy accumulate in areas where blood flow and new bone formation are increased. It is not capable of distinguishing between benign and malignant disease. Therefore, if scintigraphy shows evidence of abnormality, it has to be followed by radiography and possibly computer tomography or NMR. The sensitivity of scintigraphy to primary tumors and metastases depends on the degree of new bone formation, the individual growth rate and the blood supply. Thyroid carcinoma and multiple myeloma for example rarely have a high uptake.

Imaging techniques

Introduction

A great variety of spinal imaging techniques have become available for the detailed examination of the various structures of the lumbar spine. In many instances, these studies will provide very little additional useful information to that obtained from a thoughtful analysis of the history and physical examination. Most of these techniques employ radiation in doses which can be significant, especially to the gonads. Therefore, the physician must select the appropriate time for obtaining studies and limit the studies to those that are deemed necessary and sufficient to obtain answers to relevant clinical questions.

Plain radiographs

These studies may demonstrate a wide variety of pathological states including tumor, infection, fracture, congenital malformations, developmental abnormalities (e.g., scoliosis and spondylolisthesis), Schmorl's node, inflammatory diseases, metabolic diseases, and degenerative diseases. Plain radiographs will not demonstrate soft tissue lesions such as disc herniations or the source of a nerve root entrapment. Furthermore, pathological states such as degenerative disc disease or malalignment of facets which, in their more advanced stages, are found on these plain radiographs may not be the source of the patient's complaint as many such conditions may remain asymptomatic for a lifetime.

When it has been determined that plain radiographs are necessary for the proper study of an individual clinical situation, one must then decide which views will give the necessary information. It is wrong to use the same radiographic series for each clinical situation. An anterior-posterior view, a lateral view, and a 30 degree superiorly angled spot anterior-posterior view of the lumbosacral junction is the minimum study in most instances (Figs. 16, 17, and 18). In some patients, oblique views are necessary to demonstrate facet injuries and defects in the pars interarticularis; these are most often of value in younger patients. When it is necessary to evaluate a deformity radiographs should be taken with the patient upright and in instances of adolescent scoliosis long films will be needed. When there is a question of segmental instability active flexion-extension lateral views may have a place. Tomograms will improve the evaluation of spine fractures and infectious diseases, but has nowadays been largely replaced by CT (and/or MRI).

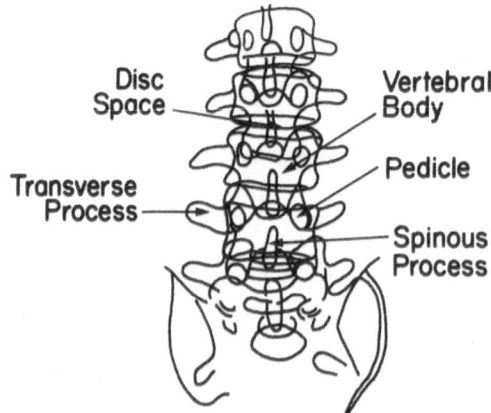

Fig. 16. A-P view of the lumbar spine

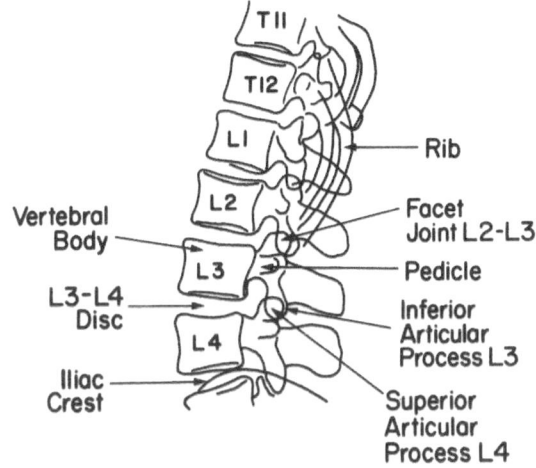

Fig. 17. Lateral view of the lumbar spine

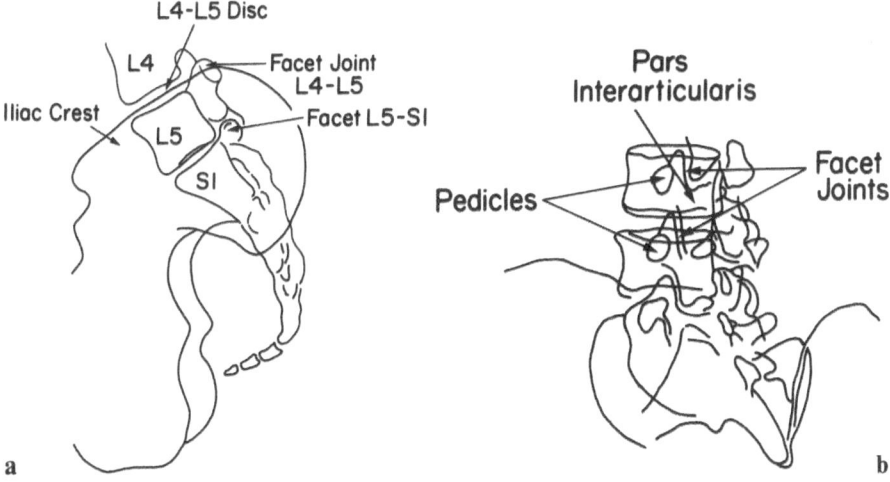

a   b

Fig. 18a Spot-lateral view of the lumbar spine. **b** Oblique view of the lumbar spine

Systematic review of film

The clinical physician who cares for patients with lumbar spine complaints should review each of the radiographic studies requested for his or her patients, not just rely on a radiographic report. Each lumbar spine film should be examined in a systematic manner. They should be placed on a source of adequate back light. The name and date should be noted as it is not uncommon to find that the wrong films are being viewed. The soft tissues should be observed next with special attention to the psoas shadows, kidneys, and great vessels. The overall alignment of the spine along with an estimate of the bone density should be observed. Lastly, the anatomy of each vertebra should be inspected in detail noting disc, pedicles, lamina, body, facets, and processes.

Findings of questionable significance

Some findings have little or no clinical significance. These include: spina bifida occulta, variations in number of lumbar vertebrae, transitional vertebrae, rudimentary ribs, Schmorl's nodes, and lordosis of less than 70°.

Findings of possible significance

Some radiographic findings may or may not be of significance in an individual case. Degenerative disease of the discs and facets are common and the incidence increases with age. They should be noted but they may not be the cause of the clinical condition being investigated. Likewise spondylolysis is often asymptomatic. Deformities such as scoliosis may not be of relevance in back pain patients while isolated vertebral tilting of slight degree may indicate the level of a discal herniation. Spondylolisthesis is often asymptomatic and so its importance in an individual instance requires clinical judgment.

Findings of definite significance

Radiographic findings indicative of tumor, infection, inflammatory disease, metabolic disease, and fracture are of urgent importance. Careful attention must be given to any areas of localized bone destruction or discontinuity which might be caused by tumor, infection, or trauma. Localized areas of increased bone density may indicate conditions as diverse as Paget's disease or metastatic carcinoma. Erosion of a pedicle indicates a slowly growing neoplasm of the spinal canal while short pedicles may indicate developmental stenosis. More subtle findings such as erosions of the sacroiliac joint, square shape to the vertebral bodies or bridging osteophytes may indicate one of the inflammatory spinal arthropathies. A uniform loss of density (osteopenia) may indicate osteoporosis, osteomalacia, or even myeloma.

Myelography

A myelogram is a radiographic study in which radio-opaque dye is instilled into the thecal sac by injection and then X-rays are obtained. Today the dyes are water soluble and rapidly excreted. They are not ionized and thus are not likely to cause hypersensitivity reactions. However, they can rarely cause significant headache, neck stiffness, nausea and vomiting, and the radiation dose necessary to complete the study is significant. Therefore, myelograms should only be done when there is suspicion of nerve involvement. The study is only of value when significant nerve root or cauda equina compression is suspected as in instances of disc hernia, spinal stenosis, and space occupying lesion such as tumor or infection. If surgical treatment is contemplated the importance of the myelogram increases significantly. In our practice myelograms are done only on patients in whom surgery is contemplated, should the study be significant.

The myelogram has some significant technical limitations: (1) In patients with severe degenerative disease it may be very difficult to place the needle in the thecal sac; (2) Myelography will not demonstrate lateral disc herniations or neuroforamenal stenosis; (3) Large L5-S1 discs may be missed in instances in which the thecal sac is normally placed posteriorly (a wide space anterior to the theca).

Computerized tomography (CT scan)

The value of CT in clinical medicine reaches beyond its considerable value in the diagnosis of individual patient problems. CT has transformed medical thought on the subject of spinal stenosis, especially with respect to the lateral nerve root entrapment syndromes, because CT allows accurate visualization of the soft tissues which are never seen well with either plain radiographs or myelography (Figs. 19 and 20). The combination of intrathecal contrast (myelography) and CT has further increased the ability to visualize morbid anatomy. CT also allows visualization of the facet joints (Fig. 21).

The difficulties with CT are three: (1) The technology is expensive and the individual studies are time consuming, increasing the cost of each study; (2) The radiation dose for each study is significant (about 5 rads); (3) The plethora of information obtained places an even greater demand on clinical judgment. These problems require that the treating physician exercise careful judgment in both the decision with respect to which patient is subjected to the study and how the study is interpreted. Much of the morbid anatomy that is found on CT has little or no relevance in an individual patient. In each case the final decision must rest on clinical grounds; the technology remains mindless.

Magnetic resonance imaging (MR scan)

This technology produces images of a form which is very much like CT. Here, however, the comparison stops as the frequency of the radiation used (within the electromagnetic spectrum) does not produce ionization in human tissues and therefore has little risk of long term deleterious effect. This is a distinct advantage over the imaging techniques so far discussed. In addition to this

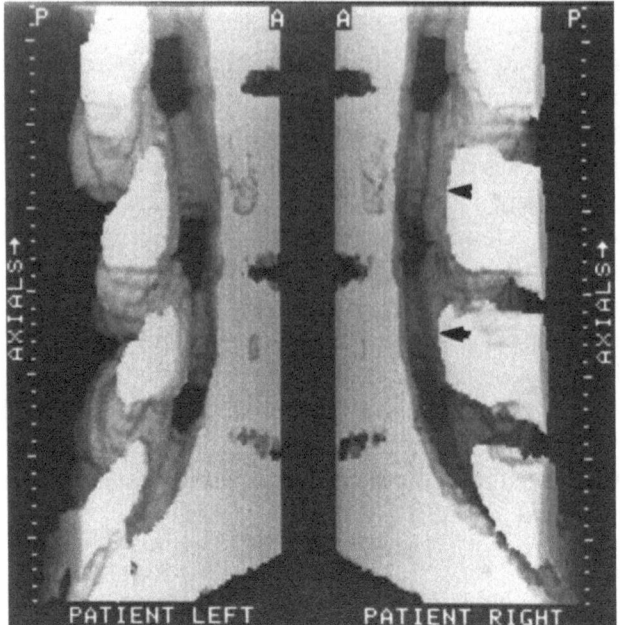

Fig. 19. CT 3-dimensional sagittal view of lumbar spine with congenital vertebral canal stenosis. Arrows indicate areas of narrowing centrally. The lateral recesses and neuroforamena are normal

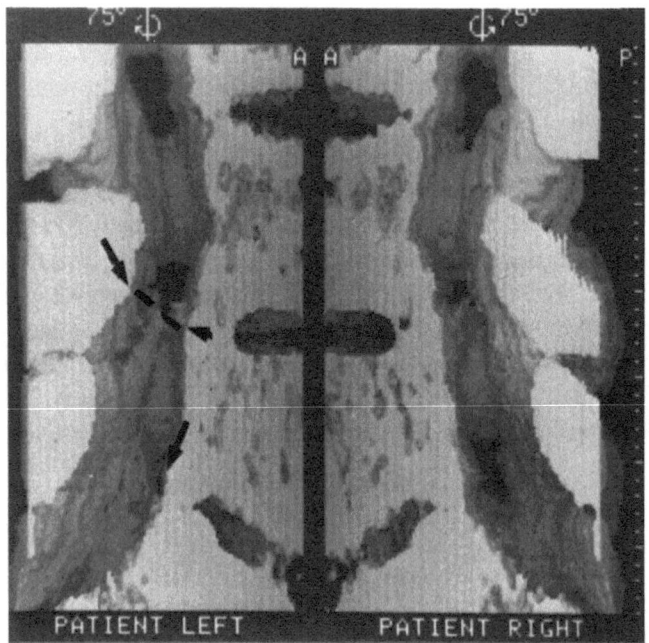

Fig. 20. Acquired vertebral canal osseous stenosis. CT 3-dimensional sagittal views, projected both to the left and right along the central axis of the canal. The stenosis of L4-5 is along an oblique plane as shown by arrows and dash line. The lower arrow identifies an osseous stenosis of the left L5-S1 neuroforamen

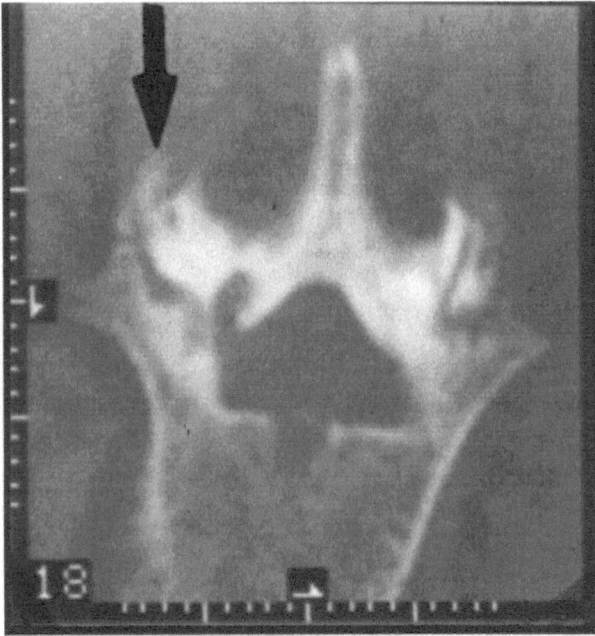

Fig. 21. Posterior facet degenerative arthritis. Axial CT section of a lumbar vertebra in the prone position. Bone hypertrophy, sclerosis, irregularity, and cystic destruction (arrow) exemplifies the severity of the arthritis

advantage, MRI provides images of soft tissue including marrow contents, disc, and intrathecal contents without the need of contrast dye or injection of radionucleides. Thus, in some instances, its use can obviate the need for myelography, CT, discography or bone scans (Fig. 22). The MRI is capable of demonstrating tumors, infection, disc degeneration, and even tears in the annulus fibrosis. It is capable of investigating the spinal cord directly.

The disadvantages of MR are many and must not be discounted. First, it is not readily available everywhere. Secondly, it is a very large and very expensive machine which takes a long time to produce an image. Thirdly, disc pathology is exaggerated and bony pathology is underestimated in many cases. Experience does not yet allow separating of useful from useless information. For a complete understanding of an individual clinical problem MR alone is frequently insufficient. Therefore, this study should only be done in very selected instances when it is most likely to provide an answer to a specific clinical question.

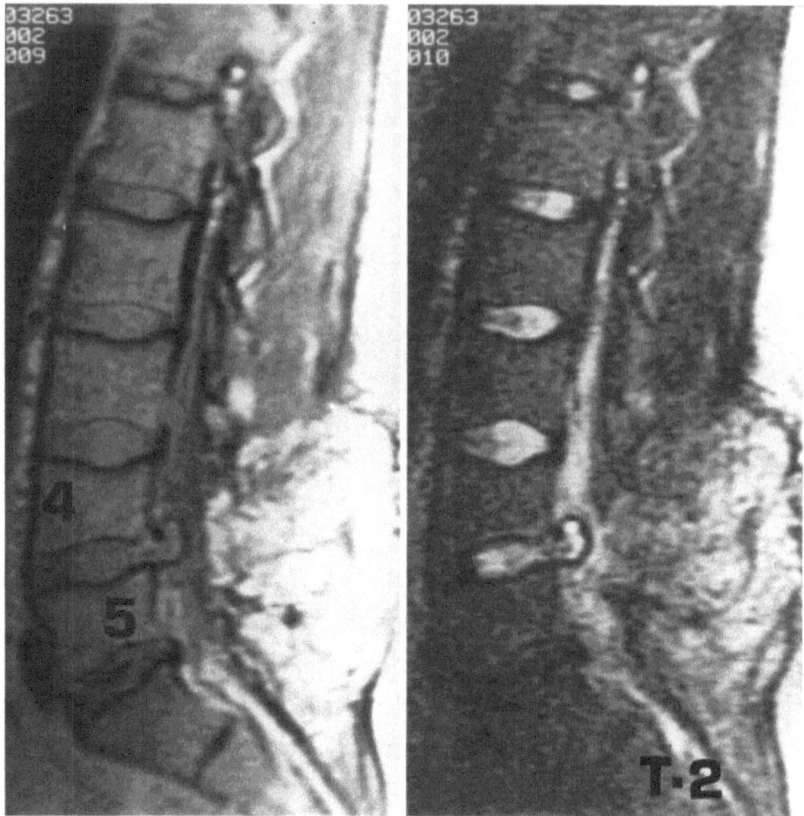

Fig. 22. Acute disc herniation MR (TR 2000/TE 20 : TR 2000/TE 70) sagittal view of the lumbar spine. The L 4-5 interspace is not dehydrated but displaced posterior with bright disc material within the vertebral canal on the T 2 image. This was an acute recurrent post (–) operative disc herniation

Which imaging technique to use when?

The choice between the different imaging procedures is not always simple. Obviously the goal is to perform that particular procedure which will best help assess the patient's problem. Most patients with low back pain do not benefit significantly from any imaging technique.

Plain films are easy to obtain and comparatively inexpensive. The bony structures can be well visualized and some information can be obtained about the state of the discs and the facet joints.

Computerized tomography delineates the bony element much better than plain films and three-dimensional reformatting allows not only axial scans (which plain films do not) but also sagittal and coronal scans. Soft tissues are visualized allowing diagnoses of disc herniations, spinal stenosis and some soft tissue masses. Radiation doses are comparatively high, however, and the cost and availability are other negative factors. Myelographic contrast can be used with CT to allow visualization of nerve roots and the spinal cord.

Myelography allows evaluation of the surface of the spinal cord and nerve roots within the thecal sac and out to the pedicle. Extradural defects in that region can therefore be detected. The cost of myelography is comparable to CT. Side effects include headaches, nausea and vomiting but are nowadays rare with the use of the modern water soluble contrast material.

Radionucleid scintigraphy is useful for early detection of bone disease, tumors and infections. It is moderate in cost and only a small amount of radiation is involved.

Magnetic resonance imaging is currently expensive and has limited availability outside the U.S. Its main benefit is that it is non-invasive and harmless. It allows direct investigation of the spinal cord. Bone marrow distortion (from tumors, infection, and trauma) is also well visualized as are degenerative disc changes and soft tissue tumors.

Plain films is the procedure of choice in trauma with CT being the next step in evaluation. MRI is an excellent procedure to evaluate sequelae of spinal cord injuries. When distinguishing between an old and a new fracture, bone scans are quite helpful.

Disc pathology is poorly visualized on plain films except in advanced stages. CT allows definition of the disc and often diagnosis of HNP and spinal stenosis. Myelograms are helpful when the CT diagnosis is uncertain. MRI is the best diagnostic method for disc degeneration, while it is not yet quite proven with respect to disc herniations and spinal stenosis. Clearly it offers an alternative to the CT.

Inflammatory diseases appear late on plain X-rays. MRI is the method of choice in infectious disease. In ankylosing spondylitis, bone scans and CT of the sacro-iliac joints, will allow early diagnoses compared to X-rays.

Tumors should first be evaluated using plain films and then those studies be supplemented by CT or MRI. MRI allows better evaluation of spinal canal extension of the mass. Bone scans are excellent screening tools because of sensitivity to early disease and because they allow the whole body to be visualized at the same time.

Measurement of bone mineral content

Plain radiographs are of limited value in determining the mineral content of bone and thus are not really useful in patients with suspected or confirmed osteoporosis. This is because the skeletal mass must be reduced by at least 30% before the loss is apparent on X-ray films and also because quantification is difficult.

Three methods are currently used: Single photon absorptiometry, dual photon absorptiometry, and quantitative computerized tomography (QCT). The single photon absorptiometry method is the one most readily available and is also comparatively inexpensive. It cannot be used for direct measurements of the spine, however, Therefore its use depends on how well cortical bone resorption mirrors cancellous bone resorption. Early stages of vertebral osteoporosis will be undetected by this method because of a lag in time between cortical bone resorption and cancellous bone resorption in osteoporosis. The use of single photon technique, therefore, is limited to patients with established osteoporosis where it can be used in follow-up of treatment.

Dual photon absorptiometry, while not yet widely available, does permit measurement in the vertebral column. Because osteophytes are often included, false values (too high) can be obtained in patients with spinal arthritis.

QCT is readily available, accurate and reproducible. The radiation dose is significant, however (500–900 mRad), and the cost high. Further, marrow fat content can lead to overestimation of bone loss.

Quantitative measurements of bone mineral contents are useful only to direct treatment. It is not a method to be used without discrimination (Chap. 16).

3 Treatment modalities

Treatment of low back pain and sciatica remains empirical. In this chapter different modalities will be reviewed and their values discussed. Specifics on when to use the treatment alternatives will be further discussed in the appropriate chapters.

Broadly, treatment can be divided into operative and non-operative (or conservative). Operative techniques will not be discussed here in detail, only to indicate what they consist of. Several textbooks describe operative treatment techniques (Rothman and Simeone, 1975; Watkins and Collis, 1987; White et al., 1987). Conservative treatment is conservative only in the sense that it does not involve an operation. In reality, conservative treatment is often more time-consuming and work-intense than operative treatment, and, in addition, can be as expensive. Recent literature reviews of various non-surgical therapies focus on their (lack of) scientific foundation (Deyo, 1983; Weber and Burton, 1986; Spitzer et al., 1987). It is obvious from these reviews that scientific evaluation of the therapeutic efficiency of many methods is either missing or inadequate. In a careful review of 721 publications only 10% were classified as scientifically "very good" (Spitzer et al., 1987). Although it is obviously unsatisfactory that science is lacking, this should not prevent us from providing therapy to our patients. Rather it should inspire to document our attempts and not use therapies with potentially harmful side effects without due attention. Nor should we treat patients for prolonged periods of time using one method, when response is slow or lacking.

Conservative (non-operative) treatment

The different conservative treatment modalities can be divided into five main categories: oral drugs, injected drugs, physical treatment methods, counter stimulation, and others.

Oral drugs

Oral drugs used in the treatment of back disorders include analgesics, non-steroidal anti-inflammatory drugs (NSAIDs), muscle relaxants, and anti-depressants. Medication is the most frequently prescribed treatment method for low back pain and sciatica. To avoid favoring of specific products only generic names are used here.

Because patients have pain, analgesics are often the first choice. Pain relief is the most obvious and concrete goal of low back pain therapy. While there are several clinical trials reported, few are technically well done and, therefore, the choice between drugs is difficult to rationalize scientifically (Deyo, 1983). The pain-relieving effect of aspirin, acetaminophen, propoxyphene hydrochloride, codeine and oxycodone are well established, however. Thus, the choice depends on severity of pain, individual response, and side effects. In general, narcotics should, and can, be avoided. Most patients respond to aspirin and acetaminophen derivates, which should be the cornerstones of the conservative treatment.

More controversial than the use of pure analgesics is whether muscle relaxants are useful adjuncts or not. Muscle relaxants, such as cariosprodol, cyclobenzaprine, methocarbamol, and diazepam are given to reduce muscle spasms associated with acute low back pain. The dosage as prescribed probably mainly induces sedation, however, while the actual muscle relaxation is minimal. Further, muscle spasms are difficult to diagnose and may, in many cases, not even exist. Side effects include drowsiness, sedation, and dizziness. In our opinion, muscle relaxants are rarely indicated, and then only for a short period.

NSAIDs, some of which are listed in Table 1, are used to reduce the inflammatory component of the patient's problem. In addition, an analgesic effect can be assumed. In our opinion, these drugs are most effective when the patient presents with an acute injury and when sciatica is present, while it is difficult to rationalize their use in chronic low back pain. Selecting the appropriate NSAID poses a problem. In 1984, there were more than a dozen NSAIDs in the U.S. and some forty-four available in Finland. Figure 1 classifies them on the basis of their chemical structure. The choice is largely empiric since there is little evidence that one is more effective than another. Nor is there evidence that combinations are more useful than single drug therapy. The older, more traditional NSAIDs have excellent anti-inflammatory effects, but side effects are more common. The newer are somewhat better tolerated. Individual response to different NSAIDs differs markedly and cannot be predicted, as does the dose response, especially in the elderly. Treatment benefits to NSAIDs are apparent in a few days. Because the half-life of NSAIDs varies greatly (from 2–96 hours), careful attention to dosages and administration is needed.

The side effects of NSAIDs include gastric irritation, anticoagulation, renal and hepatic toxicity, skin reactions and rashes, headaches, and confusion, and rarely bone marrow toxicity. Gastric irritation is quite common, supporting a recommendation to take medication with food. The anticoagu-

Table 1. Selected NSAIDs with suggested dosages and half-life

Drug	Dose range (mg/day)	Half-life (h)
Carboxylic acids		
salicylates		
acetyl salicylic acid	1000–6000	4–15
salicyl salicylate	1500–5000	4–15
indoleacetic acids		
indomethacin	50– 200	3–11
sulindac	300– 400	16
phenylalkanoic acids		
ibuprofen	1200–3200	2
ketoprofen	100– 400	2
suprofen	800	2– 4
naproxen	250–1500	13
fenamic acids		
meclofenamate	200– 400	2– 3
Pyrazoles		
phenylbutazone	200– 800	40–80
Oxicams		
piroxicam	20	30–86

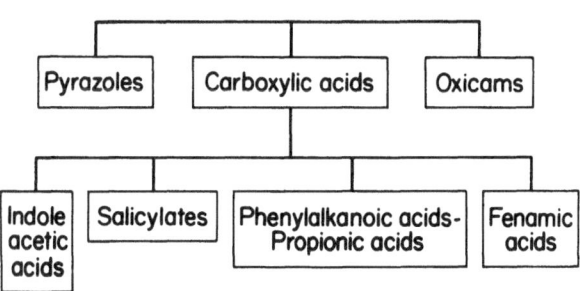

Fig. 1. Chemical classes of non-steroidal anti-inflammatory and analgesic drugs. (Adapted from Kantor, 1984)

lant effect is important should surgery be considered. To avoid excessive bleeding, aspirin medication should be stopped two weeks preoperatively while other NSAIDs need only be stopped long enough to allow their complete excretion. Some of the complications are more frequent with one chemical class of NSAIDs than with another. For example, headaches are more common with indomethacin, confusion with indomethacin, naproxen and ibuprofen and tinnitus and hearing loss with salicylates.

Oral steroids are sometimes used, particularly in patients with sciatica. The risk/benefit ratio of oral steroids on these indications is doubtful. Forty to fifty mg of prednisone orally over a 3-day period probably does not carry a high risk of complications and can be useful in the initial stages of a sciatic problem.

Tricyclic antidepressants have been shown to be effective in treating chronic low back pain with and without depression. The mechanism by which this is accomplished remains unclear. A serotonin release and compensation for a serotonin deficit has been suggested, as has a direct effect on endogenous opiate systems. Reduced anxiety and relief of muscle spasm are other possible explanations, as is relief of masked depression. In a recent study, Ward (1987) used a known comparatively selective serotonin releaser fenfluramine (40 mg) before tricyclic treatment and found that the response to treatment could be predicted based on the fenfluramine response. In the same study, CSF beta-endorphine levels were not found to change after treatment, while anxiety improved significantly. Depression was found to have a mild predictive value. This study supports the idea that the serotonin release mechanism is the important one. More importantly, however, it may be possible to predict response to tricyclic treatment using the fenfluramine test.

Injected drugs

Injected drugs should be reserved for more specific indications than oral drugs. They include parenteral corticosteroids, epidural steroids, epidural morphine, epidural anesthetics, facet joint injections, local anesthetics, and intradiscal chymopapain.

Generally, the same concerns apply to parenteral corticosteroids as to oral; they have a doubtful risk/benefit ratio.

Epidural injections have become more popular in recent years. While the use of epidural morphine and epidural anesthetics primarily aims at control of postoperative or chronic pain, epidural steroids are used both in the treatment of acute herniated lumbar discs and in spinal stenosis. It appears that results in acutely herniated discs are doubtful, while the results in spinal stenosis can be quite satisfying. Variable results can be expected, however, and the use of these injections remains controversial. Generally, epidural steroid injections are given either once, or in series of three, in which case 100–120 mgs are injected the first time and 80 mgs the second and the third time. This injection series can be repeated after a six-month interval. An anesthetic is usually injected at the same time as the steroids.

The effect of local anesthetics injected into the erector spinae muscle, or into trigger points in that muscle group, or into other muscles has not been tested properly to allow conclusions as to their efficacy. Infiltrations of this kind are done to reduce pain, and sometimes cortisone is also injected to induce an antiinflammatory effect.

Facet joint injections (or lumbar facet blocks) were introduced subsequent to the introduction of treatment methods of the so called "facet syndrome" (Ghormley, 1933; Mooney and Robertson, 1976). These treatment methods included percutaneous transections of the nerve supply to the facet joint (Rees, 1974), and percutaneous radiofrequency coagulation of these nerves (Shealy, 1976). Facet joint injections can be done for diagnostic or treatment purposes. A 22 gauge, spinal needle is directed into the joint under fluoroscopic control. Although sometimes this can be done with the patient prone, it is often best done with the patient prone but in a shallow oblique position with the affected side up. When the needle is in the joint its position can be confirmed using 0.5 cc of a water soluble contrast agent. An anesthetic and a corticosteroid can then be injected for treatment (e.g., 1.0 cc bupivacaine hydrochloride and 40 mg of methyl prednisolone acetate). For diagnostic purposes only the anesthetic is required.

Intradiscal chymopapain is being used as a treatment method for herniated lumbar discs, so called chemonucleolysis. Clinical trials have shown that chymopapain is superior to a placebo alternative with a success rate of 70% or better (Nordby, 1983; McCulloch, 1980, 1977). In studies comparing chymopapain to surgery, the surgical alternative generally gives superior short term results (Postacchini et al., 1987; Weinstein et al., 1986; Ejeskar et al., 1983). Unsuccessful chemonucleolysis allows a second line of defense, however, as surgery can be performed successfully in these patients. The main side effects of chemonucleolysis are neurologic problems which can be serious but in recent years have been rare, and anaphylaxis which occurs with an overall incidence of 0.5–1%. Efforts to reduce these side effects include a more controlled administration of the proteolytic enzyme, avoiding doing discograms at the time of injection and prescreening of patients with an IGE titer. Also, prophylactic H1 and H2 blockers as well as cortisone injections are recommended to reduce the risk of anaphylactic shock. The main remaining side effect of chemonucleolysis with chymopapain is the often reported back spasm and lower back stiffness and soreness occurring in about ¾ of the patients. After a period of initial overuse and an unacceptably high complication rate in the U.S., the enzyme treatment of herniated nucleus pulposus at this time appears to have found its role as an alternative to surgery. Additional comments on chemonucleolysis appear in Chap. 6.

Physical measures

Physical measures for conservative therapy of low back pain include bed rest, corsets, physical therapy exercises, traction, manipulation, cardiovascular exercises and the application of cold or heat. These alternatives are some-

times used in combinations and frequently also combined with an education-
al program.

Bed rest has long been the initial treatment for acute low back pain and/or
sciatica. In addition to providing symptomatic relief, a study by Wiesel et al.
(1980) shows that bed rest results in a quicker recovery at least in patients
with acute problems. Although some criticism can be voiced of this study on
military recruits, it still suggests that there is a positive effect of strict bed rest
in terms of the length of recovery. In a recent study by Deyo et al. (1987), the
optimum duration of bed rest was studied and found to be 2–3 days in a
group of patients with low back pain of nonspecific origin. Long term bed
rest has several deleterious effects and should be avoided (Waddell, 1987;
Nachemson, 1983). Medically bed rest contributes to demineralization of
bone, loss of muscle strength, decreased physical fitness, psychological distress and depression and increasing difficulty to start rehabilitation. Socially
it has negative economic consequences with loss of work habit and as time
progresses decreasing probability of returning to work. Thus, bed rest should
only be advised with acute pain, and then only for a short period. There is
no evidence that bed rest in a hospital is in any way superior to bed rest at
home, although technically rest can more easily be accomplished. The best
rest position is the so called Trendelenburg position with support under the
lower legs and with the hips and knees flexed (Fig. 2). Brief periods of sitting,
for meals, should be allowed as should the use of the bathroom. There is no
evidence that the softness of the sleeping surface is important, only that it
should not be uneven in its support of the body thus creating a hammock
situation.

Corsets and braces provide a different type of rest and are used widely.
Their superiority to placebo has not been proven but it is known that patients
who once have used a corset have a tendency to again use the corset when

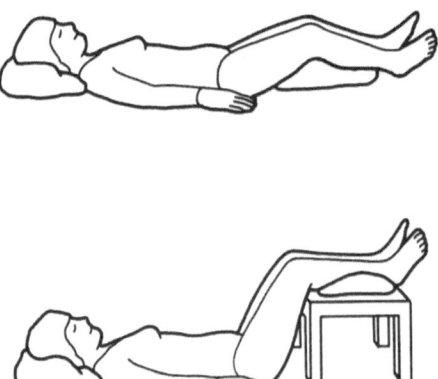

Fig. 2. The preferred rest position is lying on the back with the hips and knees flexed
(Semi-Fowler position or Trendelenburg position)

they have a recurrent attack (Ahlgren and Hansen, 1978). In chronic patients, a dependence on corsets may actually develop. There is a wide variety of corsets available from small elastic supports to high-backed corsets with metal stays. Braces are made of more sturdy materials and often require custom fitting (and molding). Several efforts have been made to study the mechanical effects of corsets and braces. Motion is restricted when a rigid brace is used but not with less rigid supports. Back muscle activity seems to be mildly affected. The intraabdominal pressure is also only mildly affected, except with certain special braces molded to that purpose. In studies of intradiscal pressures (Nachemson et al., 1983) lumbar spine compression was found to decrease in flexion but not in upright postures. In the same study no effect was noted on the intraabdominal pressure, even when a flexion jacket was used. To our mind one of the main effects of the corset is to remind the subject not to perform movements rapidly and not to flex and rotate the spine. In addition some support in upright postures can be expected. The use of corsets and braces should not be a routine treatment for patients with low back pain. Further, it should always be emphasized that they should be used short term to avoid weakening of the muscles and dependence.

The use of physical therapy in the treatment of low back pain is also common. There are four dominating classes of exercises recommended, flexion exercises (Williams, 1965), hyperextension exercises (McKenzie, 1981), general mobilizing exercises, and isometric abdominal and erector spinae muscle strengthening exercises. None of these methods has been properly evaluated, although a small study by Kendall and Jenkins (1968) appears to show an advantage of flexion exercises over general mobilizing exercises and extension exercises. Recent studies comparing McKenzie's exercises to Williams' exercises or to traction favor the McKenzie program. Further careful analysis of that concept is needed, however. Exercises performed to increase the mobility of the spine (flexion and extension exercises) place large loads on the spine (Nachemson and Elfstrom, 1970). They should therefore be avoided in the acute stages of back pain. Prophylactic back exercises to prevent future attacks and build "a muscle corset" are conceptually attractive but unproven as to their effect.

Traction has been used in the treatment of spinal disorders since prehistoric times. Various types of traction can be applied, such as intermittent traction, heavy or light traction, auto traction and traction with the spine in a number of different postures. The physiological mechanisms of why traction can be effective is unclear. The disc space can increase following traction, and the lumbar lordosis often decreases. Epidurograms and myelograms have shown that a disc protrusion can be reduced. Disc pressure studies (Andersson et al., 1983) indicate that with passive traction pressure decreases can be obtained, while with active (so called autotraction) the pressure increases. In the short term muscle activity tends to increase while after a period a decrease can occur. Other theories are that the mechanoreceptors of the back are affected, or that muscle spasm is reduced. To actually accomplish spinal traction a force of 25 % or more of the body has to be applied, because of friction. This means that the pelvic traction sometimes applied to patients over a long period with 10 kg (20 lb) weights only serves the purpose of keeping the patient in bed. Several therapeutic trials of traction have been performed. In at least one of these (Larson et al., 1980) auto-traction was found to be superior to the use of a corset at one week, but not at three-months following treatment application. Auto-traction is a technique in which the patient's pelvis is fixed to a frame and then the patient applies a force by pulling with the arms. The patient's posture can be adjusted in three planes. In a subsequent study by Ljunggren et al. (1984) comparing auto-traction to manual placebo traction in patients with sciatica, no difference in efficiency was found. The most frequently used form of traction is intermittent lumbar traction. Traction is put on the pelvis for up to 30 minutes in intermittent periods and with loads up to 75 kg. Other types of traction such as gravity traction and the use of gravity boots have been advocated by some but have not yet been scientifically tested.

Manipulation is highly controversial, in part because there is no clear biological rationale and, in part because randomized trials have come to conflicting results. While there is no doubt that manipulation is effective in some patients, it remains to be shown in whom and to what degree it is superior to a placebo alternative. Further there are numerous manipulative techniques in current use making the issue even more complex. For more information on clinical trials of manipulation please refer to Buerger and Greenman (1984), Graham (1980), and Dixon et al. (1985). Manipulation does not usually result in immediate freedom of pain, although this has been described. Further in some patients no effect at all is obtained. It appears that at best manipulation can reduce the period of painful disability in some patients (Hadler et al., 1987). Mobilization aims at stretching or rupturing micro- or macro-adhesions in the facet joints and other spinal structures. It

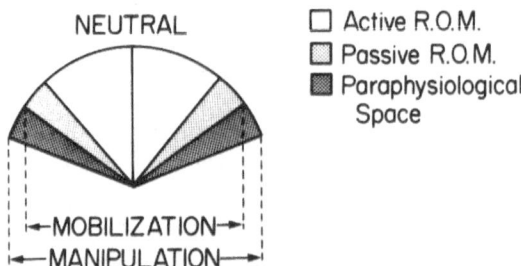

Fig. 3. Joint mobilization means passive motion up to the barrier of resistance, while manipulation is a forced movement beyond usual physiological limits. (Adapted from Buerger and Greenman, 1985)

is a different procedure from manipulation in that the movement is "controlled", while in manipulation a high-velocity thrust is made which is not controllable once initiated (Fig. 3). There is no scientific support to mobilization at the present time although in some patients increased mobility can be documented following treatment.

Local application of heat or cold results in dramatic relief in some patients, while others find the modalities unacceptable. Again, there is no clear knowledge about in whom and at what point these treatment methods would be advisable. It appears that in the acute stages, cold treatment (10–20 minutes if a cold pack is used) can have some pain-relieving effect, perhaps by providing counter-stimulation. Inflammation and edema subsequent to acute injury can be reduced by cooling. Heat provided as a heating pad or similar does not penetrate the skin and subcutaneous tissue, yet can induce a feeling of reduced pain, perhaps by increasing the pain threshhold. This can be beneficial before exercise therapy, manipulation or traction. Heat should not be used in treatment of an acute injury since its application can increase edema and thereby pressure on the nociceptors. Any relief from these modalities is transient.

Short wave diathermy (SWD) is another method used to treat patients with low back pain. SWD is a method where a high-frequency current is converted into heat in the tissues. It is supposed to penetrate more deeply than superficial heat. A thorough scientific evaluation of this treatment still awaits us. However, SWD, has been tested against manipulation and in one study (Gibson et al., 1985) also against placebo. In that study neither manipulation nor SWD was found to be more effective than placebo.

Massage and ultrasound (very high frequency waves used to provide "deep heat") are other treatment modalities that are sometimes used in the treatment of soft tissue low back injuries. Neither stands up to a scientific scrutiny and should definitely only be used short term to improve subjective comfort. A desirable effect is usually evident in the first or second session. Long term use of these modalities have a negative effect as they tend to pacify the patients.

Counter stimulation

Counter stimulation includes the use of transcutaneous electrical nerve stimulation (TENS, TNS), acupuncture and various types of implantable neurostimulators. TENS is a high-frequency sensory stimulation using pulsed current.

The use of TENS is based on the gate control theory which proposes that pain perception can be modulated by altering the sensory input. By stimulating the large sensory afferent nerves nociceptive stimulation is closed out. While there are no randomized clinical trials in low back patients, there appears to be some pain relieving effect from the use of TENS. An advantage of TENS is that it is self-administered and can be used to replace medication. The electrodes are either placed in the area of pain or in its dermatomal distribution. Acupuncture, on the other hand, has been tested against other treatment modalities and has not proven to be superior to placebo. Implanted neurostimulators have their limited place in the treatment of chronic, unbearable low back pain.

Other types of non-operative treatment

Biofeedback, back schools and behaviorial therapy are other treatment modalities used for low back pain and sciatica. While biofeedback and behaviorial therapy are primarily used in the treatment of chronic, unrelenting pain, back schools have been used for the purpose of providing prophylaxis and recovery during periods of acute and chronic low back pain. Back schools provide an important adjunct to other types of conservative treatment methods. Generally they include information on anatomy, physiology and function of the spine as well as on body mechanics and preventive back care. The natural course of low back pain is explained and treatment principles are outlined. Back schools are not a substitute for other types of treatment, however. They will improve patient understanding and make the patients aware of their responsibilities in managing their spine problems.

Operative treatment

Surgery in low back pain and sciatica is primarily performed for disc herniations, spinal stenosis, spondylolisthesis, and so called spinal instability. In addition, surgery is also performed for tumors and infections which are rare, and for spinal deformity and trauma. Surgery in not indicated for "idiopathic low back pain" and generally should be used only when other treatment modalities fail. A demonstrable, precisely diagnosed structural lesion should be present.

The most common approach to the lumbar spine is a posterior approach through a longitudinal incision in the midline. This provides direct access to the spinous processes, laminae and facet joints at all levels of the lumbar spine. The transverse processes can also be reached by retracting the paraspinal muscles laterally. By removing ligament and/or bone from the laminae and retracting the dura, the disc space can be reached. A postero-lateral approach has been described as an alternative to expose the transverse processes. Following a midline skin incision the incision of the fascia is made lateral and then the dissection is carried down between the sacrospinal and transversospinal muscles. Because less muscle mass has to be retracted medially, exposure of the facet joints is easier with less blood loss (Wiltse, 1968). An antero-lateral approach allows exposure of the lumbar vertebral bodies for purposes such as infection drainage, biopsies, anterior resections and anterior fusion.

A *laminotomy* means removal of a small part of the lamina, i.e., for the purpose of removing a herniated nucleus pulposus. This procedure is sometimes also referred to as fenestration or interlamilar exploration, and often involves removing small amounts of both the superior and inferior lamina (Fig. 4).

In recent years, the use of a microscope or magnifying glasses in disc hernia surgery has become increasingly common. This procedure, sometimes referred to as *microscopic discectomy,* and sometimes as limited exposure discectomy improves visualization of the area allowing a relatively less traumatic dissection, using a smaller incision. Recovery subsequent to the operation, therefore, is quicker. The procedure does require a high degree of skill and training, however, and failures can occur due to retained disc fragments not observed through the keyhole approach. The conventional disc excision also requires minimal, if any, bone resection. For patients with proper indication a short term success rate, from 90–95% can be expected. The disc is, of course, never removed in its entity but only those parts that can be easily extracted through the limited incision in the posterior annular wall.

Transcutaneous disc surgery or *percutaneous discectomy* is a relatively new technique by which an instrument is inserted from the postero-lateral route into the disc center and disc tissue is mechanically disintegrated and removed through suction. This technique must still be considered experimental, awaiting documented clinical results.

Laminectomies are frequently used in surgical treatment of spinal stenosis. This procedure involves removing the lamina on one side (hemilaminectomy) (Fig. 4) or the spinous process and both laminae (wide laminectomy) (Fig. 4). The number of laminae to be removed is assessed by the preoperative structural evaluation and by what is seen at the time of the operation. Deciding how much of each lamina and how many laminae to remove is sometimes difficult. Pulsation of the dura can be used as a guide. Since following very wide laminectomies there is an increased risk of instability as

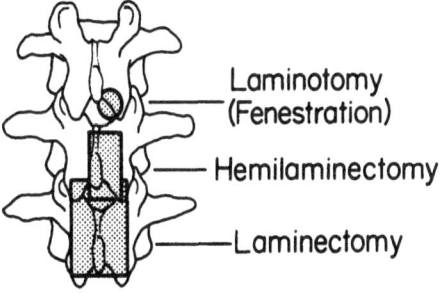

Fig. 4. Amount of bone removed in a laminotomy, a hemilaminectomy, and a (wide) laminectomy

much as possible of the posterior joints should be left intact. Enough of the articular process must be removed, however, to deal with the indentation of the dura and entrapment of the nerve in the lateral recess.

Spinal fusion is rarely indicated in the treatment of uncomplicated disc herniations, if ever. Retrospective studies comparing conventional disc excision without and with spinal fusion indicate that there is no significant benefit in terms of back pain recurrence or rate of reoperation. Spinal fusion places increases stress on adjacent disc levels, creating in the long run an increased risk for spinal stenosis. Further the morbidity is greater and postoperative pain frequently occurs in the bone graft donor area. In other conditions such as segmental instabilities, spine fusion is the operation of choice, however. Although there is considerable controversy about the term segmental instability as such, it is here used to indicate abnormal motion taking place at the motion segment level. Examples of conditions in which segmental stability can be present is spondylolisthesis and spinal trauma. It can also occur secondary to severe degenerative disc disease and to removal of posterior elements for spinal stenosis.

The most frequently used method of spinal fusion is the postero-lateral fusion, placing bone grafts over the transverse processes and lateral aspects of the facet joints. The area to be fused can be explored through the posterior incision or through the postero-lateral incision discussed above. Fusion is not always simple to accomplish. A pseudarthrosis rate of about 25% can be expected, with a greater risk of a failed fusion at higher lumbar levels. To improve on the rate of fusion, segmental spinal instrumentation has become increasingly popular. While the use of those instrumentations carries complications, there seems to be an immediate advantage in terms of post-operative recovery. Whether or not the long-term fusion rates in the hands of the average orthopaedic surgeon will be improved remains to be seen. In cases of spondylolisthesis, posterolateral fusion is usually combined with the removal of the loose part of the neural arch. In patients with degenerative "spinal instability" removal is only indicated when the neural structures are involved.

Posterior fusions can be performed when the posterior elements are left intact. In this operation, the bone grafts are placed alongside and between the spinous processes and roughened laminae as well as packed into the intervertebral joints.

Anterior fusions, often referred to as anterior interbody fusions are usually performed only when the anterior parts of the spine, for some reason, are involved in the disease process or when previous posterior and lateral fusions have failed. In patients with previous laminectomies and small transverse processes, anterior fusions may have to be performed should fusion at all be considered. In some cases of developmental spondylolisthesis anterior fusion is also indicated.

4 The patient with acute low back pain

Introduction

The twelve symptoms and signs in Table 1 constitute the most common significant clinical syndrome in the constellation of syndromes in which "acute low back pain" is the central unifying symptom. It is rare, however, that the actual patient's symptoms and signs have a one-to-one correspondence with this list. One or several of the twelve can be missing. However, significant deviations from this list should warn the clinician that a different and possibly more serious pathological condition may be present. Conversely, absolute correspondence with this list does not guarantee that the pathologies described below are the cause of the patient's symptoms. The physician must be diligent in observing the patient's changing state so as to detect changes that will require a new analysis of the patient's status and a new approach to diagnosis and treatment.

Table 1. Signs and symptoms in patients with acute low back pain

Symptoms	Signs
Sudden onset	Local spinal tenderness
Relieved by rest	Flat back
Aggravated by motion	Possible list
Radiation no lower than thigh	Spasms
Non-radicular	Limitation of spinal motion
Fetal position = comfort	
Age usually under 40	

Some of the terminology used in this chapter and in subsequent chapters of this book are not in common use in general medicine. "Overload" in our particular context is a term which refers to the application of a force to the spine which is sufficient to produce permanent deformation or outright failure of one or more of the different structural components of the back. Our choice of the term signifies our belief that mechanical factors are important, and corresponds also to a frequent description by the patient as to how the back problem originated. Typically, the overload described by the patient is sudden as in a lifting "accident". This form of overload may result in a variety of injuries such as a ligamentous or muscular strain or sprain, or bone or cartilage fracture, with associated hematoma and swelling. Other forms of failure occur as a result of "fatigue" which is the gradual development of cracks in the spinal structural materials as a result of repetitive loading, another form of overload (see Chap. 1).

"Spasm" is a term which is used to denote an involuntary muscular contraction. The spasm may be either "clonic" or "tonic". A clonic contraction is intermittent and is broken by relaxation of the involved muscle; while a tonic spasm is continuous. The usual clinical experience is that of clonic spasms which are precipitated by motion. Spasm can sometimes be seen as a "swelling", sometimes only palpated as a "hard" muscle.

Typical history

In the younger population (usually before the age of forty years) the most common low back pain syndrome is that of a rather sudden onset of severe pain, not infrequently, following an episode of overload. The patient will often describe an "accident" in which a specific moment of injury was appreciated. One typical history is that of the "lifting accident" in which the patient attempted a difficult lift of excessive weight or perhaps a quite trivial weight in an awkward posture. Occasionally, the patient will describe a surprise overload situation in which a load is being carried by two or more workers and one of them lets go of his share of the load suddenly, overloading his partner. However, a significant number of patients will not have been aware of any precipitating cause of their acute episode of low back pain. This is important to recognize; acute does not mean sudden and is usually not the result of "accident" in the usual context of that word.

The onset is often a sudden twinge of pain in the lower back, which initially may or may not be severe; however, within a few hours the back becomes progressively more painful with the sensation of increasing stiffness. By the next morning the patient is nearly unable to rise from bed and any motion will produce severe pain and "spasm" of the paraspinal muscles.

The pain is described as sharp, stabbing or cramping in nature and is tolerable if motion is avoided. The mere act of rising from bed can take many minutes and sometimes requires the help of another person. The patient may describe rolling out of bed onto his knees and pushing himself to the upright using the bed or a chair. Walking is difficult, clumsy, slow, and painful. Coughing or sneezing brings on paroxysms of pain (spasm). The pain may be in the back only, or may radiate to the region of the sacroiliac joints, upper buttocks and sometimes to one or both upper thighs or groin. The pain in acute low back pain does not radiate below the knee and is not associated with parasthesias, numbness or weakness.

Physical findings

An observation of the patient undressing is often quite revealing. These patients are frequently unable to remove their stockings and require help. The gait is guarded and slow. Normally, the shoulders and upper thorax rotate in the opposite direction from the lower spine and pelvis when walking. Patients with acute low back pain will often eliminate this rotary motion, and will rock from side to side with a flat back and a slight flexion deformity. They may sometimes present with a tilt to one side, with a postural flexion abnormality and with a functional scoliosis. The paraspinal muscles appear to be tight "hard", although EMG studies have failed to show persistent significant increases in electrical activity. There is local tenderness over the mid-line spinous processes or just lateral to the mid-line over the erector spinae muscles. The tenderness is not diffuse and not cutaneous, but deep. Deep pressure can give temporary relief of the pain and is sometimes sought by the patient. The straight leg raising test often produces back pain, but does not produce leg pain. The hamstring muscles may be tight, but motor point tenderness is absent. Loading of the shoulders and false rotation (see Chap. 2) do not significantly increase the pain, although the patient may be quite apprehensive and resist these tests out of fear. Weakness, sensory changes, and reflex changes are absent. The sacroiliac stress tests produce severe back pain and "spasm", and are therefore not possible to perform properly.

Pathologic anatomy in acute low back pain

An actual pathologic anatomical entity is rarely observed in patients with acute low back pain. However, what occurs in instances of overload can reasonably be inferred from the various laboratory studies of loads applied to cadaveric spines combined with the pathologic studies of spines at various ages. These changes have been described earlier in Chap. 1. In summary, a variety of possible injuries can occur to any of the structural elements of the spine including bone, cartilage, ligament, and muscles. Compressive overload can produce stellate fractures of the end plate with injury to the attachment of the hyaline cartilage of the end plate. Twisting overload can produce tears in the annulus fibrosis. Overload in extension can result in facet injuries; and, if the force is great enough, fractures of the pars interarticularis have been observed secondary to such trauma. Sudden muscular contraction can result in avulsion fractures of the transverse processes. Ruptures of muscle fibers or collagen tissue have not actually been observed but are quite reasonable assumptions, since they do occur in other parts of the body. Severe overloads with identifiable bony injuries, which can be seen on X-rays, are quite unusual. Patients with osteopenia can, however, sustain fractures with trivial or unrecognized trauma (see Chap. 17).

Laboratory and structural studies

The use of laboratory and structural studies must be viewed in light of the excellent prognosis of acute low back pain. Most patients recover in a three week period. Controversy surrounds the use of X-rays in these patients on their initial presentation (Chap. 2). Initially, spine radiographs in patients with acute low back pain (without significant trauma) are not necessary; and, moreover, they seldom yield useful information pertaining to the specific diagnosis. On the other hand, in instances in which the patient's syndrome deviates significantly from the "typical" situation as presented in Table 1, or when the symptoms have persisted for more than one or two weeks without significant improvement then a lumbosacral X-ray study as described in Chap. 2 is appropriate. There are good arguments for limiting the number and frequency of medical radiation studies in patients with an acute episode of lower back pain: (1) the low yield and high costs result in a low cost/benefit ratio; (2) even if the quantity of radiation in an individual study is very small it adds to the preexisting background radiation. Every effort should be made to avoid X-rays in patients who may be pregnant.

No other studies are appropriate in the assessment of the patient with acute low back pain. CT scans, MRI and electrodiagnostics are not indicated.

Treatment

The treatment of an episode of acute low back pain is entirely symptomatic in nature (see Chap. 2). The natural history of the process is persistence of symptoms for a period of one to three weeks (Fig. 1). Weisel et al. (1980) demonstrated that in a military population a course of rest in bed and acetylsalicylic acid (ASA) was an effective therapy. Deyo et al. (1986) took this further and have shown that the actual period of bed rest (after two days) has no influence on the eventual outcome of treatment. Many medications have been recommended as treatment choices for the relief of the symptoms in an acute episode of severe lower back pain. So called "muscle relaxants" are prescribed in great numbers. However, the effectiveness of these medications remains questionable. If an analgesic more potent than simple anal-

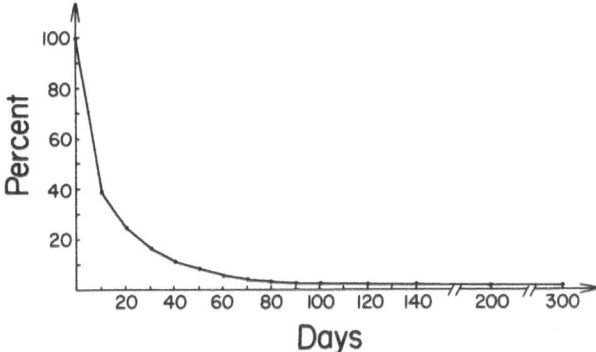

Fig. 1. Normal recovery and return to work in patients with low back pain (Adapted from Andersson et al., 1982)

gesics is required, then codeine is acceptable for short periods. The problem of dependency can only be controlled by the restriction of the number and frequency of use of the medication. Once the acute episode is over the patient should be prescribed an individually tailored program of physical exercises based upon his or her individual needs and physical status.

We recommend that the treatment for a patient with an acute episode of lower back pain should follow a specific plan. This plan of treatment is designed to achieve the goal of rapid restoration of function with the least risk of further injury and the prevention of chronic illness behavior. Upon presentation to the office, clinic, or emergency service the patient should be made comfortable to facilitate the taking of an adequate history. Time and patience are required for the physical examination to allow the patient's fears of increasing pain and spasm to subside, and to gain his/her confidence in the treatment program and future recommendations. When history and physical examinations have been completed the patient needs to be informed of the benign nature of the illness and that it is expected that most, if not all, patients are recovered sufficiently to return to moderate activity by one to three weeks and to full and unrestricted activity by six weeks. Further, the patient needs to be informed of the policy regarding radiographs, which in nontraumatic cases is to wait for radiographs until at least one week has passed without improvement in symptoms. In our opinion, however, it is important not to make this a major issue with the patient. Some patients urgently want X-ray examination and a controversy with the patient can create an unfortunate loss of confidence in suggested treatment.

The treatment for the first two days is modified bed rest in which the patient may arise for meals and to use the toilet. The position assumed should be on the side or back with the hips or knees flexed. The bed should be arranged for maximum comfort with a bolster or pillows which can be placed behind the knees to achieve the hip and knee flexed position when the patient is supine. The patient should be taught to rise without spine motion using the legs over the edge of the bed as a counterbalance. Medications for the first two days may include a small amount of codeine or similar. However, this must not be continued for more than a few days and the patient must understand the dangers of long term use of this class of medication. Non-narcotic pain relievers are to be used thereafter.

On the third day the patient begins a program of gradually increasing activity. This activity should include walking and mild back limbering exercise. The walking should be for short distances and repeated. Several walks of 500 to 1000 meters (half a mile) are adequate. The limbering exercise should begin with three gentle movements in flexion, extension, and lateral bending over only the initial one-fourth of the normal range of motion. We recommend that the patients do this before each meal (a memory device only). Each day the number of movements is increased and the range is increased. Sitting is restricted to a maximum of half an hour at a time. Driving is discouraged. The patient is instructed to report the development of significant deterioration of his/her status, including the development of sciatica or urinary retention.

The first follow-up visit is at one week. Radiographs are now obtained if there has been no significant improvement in the patient's status. As is often the case, recovery is in progress and often nearly complete and the patient can be returned to sedentary work with a program of conditioning excercises designed to control weight and promote cardiovascular fitness (Nutter, 1987). Instructions in back and abdominal strengthening exercises, in general

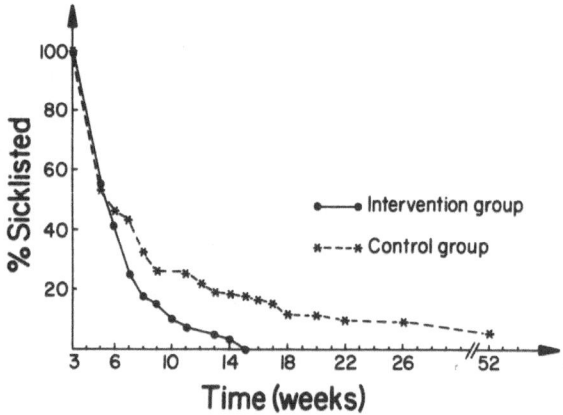

Fig. 2. Percent of patients still sicklisted at 3–52 weeks. The difference between the intervention group and the control group is highly significant (Adapted from Chöler et al., 1985)

conditioning, and in proper lifting and other back care techniques should be arranged for at a later session (often with a trained therapist, and in the form of a mini back school).

A more elaborate rehabilitation program will be necessary for patients who claim an on-the-job injury or who do heavy manual work. This program should include some formal estimate of the demands of the job and the patient's physical ability to meet these demands. When specific deficiencies are detected these should be corrected with a directed course of physical therapy or work hardening. The importance of active treatment cannot be overestimated in these patients who have an increased risk of becoming chronic low back sufferers. As shown by Chöler et al. (1985) active and well-managed treatment hastens recovery (Fig. 2). Wiesel et al. (1980) found that by instituting a treatment algorithm return to work occurs earlier with significant savings in cost. Important to the treatment of this group of patients is an understanding attitude on the side of the employer. Light duty work should be provided if at all possible.

In any patient in whom the problem of lower back pain remains, and in whom the illness lasts more than six weeks further investigations will be necessary. The problems relating to severe and unremitting lower back pain are covered in Chap. 7 while those relating to moderate chronic pain are covered in Chap. 10. A careful search for secondary gain must also begin at this point (see Chap. 13).

5 The patient with recurrent low back pain

Introduction

Recurrences are part of the natural history of low back pain. In two prospective studies of industrial populations, recurrent symptoms occurred within one year in 60 percent of those workers who had an acute low back pain episode (Bergquist-Ullman and Larsson, 1977; Troup et al., 1981). A history of sciatica has been found to indicate increased risk of recurrence (Troup et al., 1981; Biering-Sorensen, 1983). Biering-Sorensen (1983), in a prospective Danish study found that the risk of recurrent low back pain in the first year increased when there had been (1) many previous back pain episodes, (2) many previous sickness-absence days because of low back pain, (3) short intervals between previous episodes, and (4) an aggravated course of a previous episode. This indicates that the more severe the back problem, the greater the risk of recurrent episodes. Although these studies give some information about the risk of recurrent low back pain, we do not know in an individual patient how great that risk is. Nor do we know precisely how to reduce that risk.

History and physical examination

It is important to distinguish between patients who have recurrent low back pain with completely pain free episodes in between, from those with exacerbations of an ongoing pain problem. In the first case, which is the group of patients discussed in this chapter, each episode can be seen as a new acute low back pain episode, while in the second we are dealing with a chronic back problem. The acute syndromes are discussed in Chaps. 4 and 6, while the chronic syndrome will be discussed in Chap. 10. The patient with recurrent back pain presents with symptoms and signs similar to those of the patient with acute low back pain (Chap. 4) and/or acute sciatica (Chap. 6). The difference lies in the fact that the problem has occurred in the past. This past experience will significantly influence the patient's perception of his or her present problem. Therefore, it is important to obtain information about previous attacks, their course and their treatment. Rapid recovery from previous low back problems is a positive sign, indicating excellent prognosis for this episode as well. Conversely, slow recovery with prolonged sickness absence from work in a previous episode is a poor prognostic sign, and should alert the physician that this patient requires careful attention so as not to develop a chronic back problem.

Previous surgery is also important information. Does the patient's problem represent a recurrent disc prolapse? Is it a complication of previous diagnostic tests and treatments such as arachnoiditis, scar tissue formation, "instability" or abnormal stress distribution within the lumbar spine secondary to fusion and/or instrumentation? These previously operated patients present complex diagnostic and treatment problems and should be managed by someone with a special interest in low back problems. Information about the initiating event of previous and present episode(s) is also important. Work related "injuries", when occurring time after time should lead to an analysis of the patient's work situation and should raise the suspicion that there may be a mismatch between the patient's capacity and his or her work requirements. Should the workplace be addressed rather than the patient? Should a change in work be suggested? Can the patients improve on their physical capabilities by appropriate physical rehabilitation? Again, this analysis requires an interest in back pain and also that a careful work history is obtained and that a functional evaluation is performed.

Recurrent sciatica is not uncommon in patients with central disc herniations. Sometimes, then, pain will move from one leg, in a previous episode, to the other leg. More often, however, the same leg is painful in recurrent episodes.

Patients with spondylolisthesis will often have recurrent episodes. In these patients, work relatedness is not infrequent and, therefore, a work history should always be obtained.

A special subgroup of patients with recurrent problems are those with spinal stenosis (Chap. 9).

Diagnostics

Radiographs should be obtained in these patients if they do not already exist. Repeat radiographs are rarely indicated, however, and they yield limited new information. The exceptions to this basic principle are when previous radiographs are several years old, when an external injury has occurred, when significant new symptoms and signs are present and when suspicion exists that the cause may be tumor, infection or metabolic disease (see Chaps. 14, 15, and 17). As discussed elsewhere, radiographs are more often indicated in the young patient (below age 20) and in the middle aged and older patients (above age 50).

CT and MRI scans are no more indicated in patients with recurrent back problems than they are in those with acute back pain. This means that only patients in which suspicion exists of nerve compression, tumor or infection should be scanned. Myelograms are only indicated when surgery is contemplated. Bone scans and neurodiagnostics are rarely indicated in recurrent low back pain.

Functional tests of range of motion, strength and endurance are indicated when a suspicion exists that there is a mismatch between the patient's capabilities and his or her work demand.

Treatment

The goals of the treatment of patients with recurrent low back pain should be: (1) to treat the acute episode; (2) to prevent the problem from becoming chronic; and (3) to prevent new episodes from occurring. To accomplish the first goal the treatment methods discussed in Chap. 3 should be used as appropriate for patients with low back pain and low back and leg pain (Chaps. 4 and 6). Preventing the problem from becoming chronic involves active interventions following a short period of rest, with an emphasis on activity and early work return. This is discussed elsewhere in this book. Prevention of recurrent episodes, or at least reduction in rate and severity of episodes is the most important treatment message of this chapter. Unfortunately, there are no hard scientific data that recurrent episodes can be prevented, such a study would be almost impossible to accomplish. There is evidence, however, that information will help patients avoid activities and postures that are stressful to the spine and, therefore, avoid triggering low back pain. Further, information will help patients cope with problems in case they occur, thus, reducing the need for physician visits and medical treatment. In our opinion, information should be given all patients with recurrent low back pain. This information should include the natural history of low back pain, risk factors, body mechanics and self-treatment. The back school provides a convenient model to disseminate information but it is not the only method available. Books, pamphlets, and, most importantly, frank conversations with the patient can yield similar results.

Improved physical condition is another preventive method that should be employed. Patients with recurrent low back pain are sometimes fearful of exercise since they believe that this will bring back the problem. This misconception should be clarified, and the patient stimulated to improve their cardio-vascular function by swimming, rapid walking, bicycling, and jogging.

Abdominal and back muscle strengthening exercises to build up the "muscle corset" should also be encouraged, as should stretching exercises. These exercises are often best taught by a physical therapist who also should provide the patient with illustrations for review and reference at home. When a functional evaluation is done, results can be used as guidelines for functional improvement.

The use of corsets is controversial. Patients who always develop their recurrent episodes when doing unaccustomed stressful activities can do quite well by using a corset during these activities. An example is the orthopedic surgeon who develops back pain every spring when doing gardening and every fall when splitting logs, but is otherwise doing quite well. The logical advice would be not to do gardening and log splitting, but if for some reason this is unacceptable, then a corset used during these activities (and not at any other time) can be helpful.

Summary

Recurrent back pain is common and sometimes frightening to the patient. When occurring, each episode should be treated as any acute back pain episode, and then information and conditioning be initiated to prevent future recurrences, and make it easier for the patient to deal with those.

6 The patient with pain radiating down the leg

Introduction

In epidemiologic research the term "sciatica" is often used to denote pain in the leg originating from the spine. In a closer sense, however, sciatica means involvement of one of the nerve roots making up the sciatic nerve or of the sciatic nerve proper. In this chapter we will use the term "sciatica" as the symptom of pain radiating down the posterior leg to the foot or ankle in the distribution of one or several lumbar nerve roots. "Sciatica" may be associated with parasthesias, numbness, and sometimes muscular weakness leading in its extreme to muscular wasting in the leg. Pain in part of the sciatic distribution as in the buttocks or posterior thigh which does not extend below the knee is not sciatica in the sense in which it will be used in this discussion, but, rather is called "referred" pain. When numbness or weakness is present in the distribution of a specific nerve root the patient is said to have a

Table 1. Different etiologies in true sciatica and referred leg pain

Sciatica	Referred leg pain
Disc hernia	Spondylosis
Spondylosis Tumor of nerve or involving nerve	Tumor of vertebra pelvis sacrum
Infection epidural abscess vertebral infection with bony destruction	Infection vertebral pelvic SI joint
Herpes zoster or post herpetic neuralgia	Intra pelvic disease
Trauma to nerve	Tumor Abscess Endometriosis

"radiculopathy" (e.g., L-5 radiculopathy) in addition to sciatica (when pain is present).

There are many causes of sciatica including: (1) tumors of the cauda equina and other irritative intrathecal lesions; (2) herpes zoster and post herpetic neuralgia; (3) intrapelvic visceral or bony lesions directly involving the lumbosacral plexus; (4) injuries or tumors directly involving the sciatic nerve itself; and (5) diseases of the lumbar vertebra which produce a direct effect upon the cauda equina or individual nerve roots. The most common cause of sciatica before late middle age (55 +) is protrusion of the intervertebral disc producing pressure upon an individual nerve root or upon the cauda equina (Table 1).

Typical history

The syndrome outlined in Table 2 includes all of the signs and symptoms commonly seen in patients who have recently protruded (herniated) a lumbar intervertebral disc posteriorly or postero-laterally sufficiently to produce nerve compression, tension or irritation. The syndrome can appear suddenly with little or no warning and without recognized precipitating factors. However, the majority of patients will have experienced one or more episodes of lower back pain of varying intensity and duration with partial or complete recovery after a period of rest. These episodes often began years before the first episode of sciatica (see Chaps. 4 and 5).

The typical patient is a male or female in the 35 to 45 year age range who has experienced at least one significant episode of lower back pain in the past and who was well until he or she experienced a sudden "catch" or "snap"

Table 2. Typical symptoms and signs in patients with pain radiating down the leg. Patients usually present with some of these, rarely with all

Symptoms	Signs
Sudden onset of lower back pain	Flat back
Average age forty years	List
Associated leg pain radiating below the knee	"Spasm"
	Localized lumbar spinal tenderness
Associated parasthesias in the leg or foot	Limitation of spinal motion
	Positive stretch test
Lower extremity weakness	Reflex change
Lower extremity numbness	Sensory change
Aggravated by sneezing or coughing	"Lead pipe" weakness
Aggravated by sitting	Sciatic notch tenderness
Aggravated by lying on the abdomen	

in the back followed by the rather rapid onset of spasm, severe low back pain with or without sciatica, and the inability to straighten up the back. The patient often describes a seemingly trivial injury such as bending over to pick up a small object. For the first few minutes or hours pain can be moderate. The full blown lumbar portion of the syndrome is usually well established by the next morning, making it difficult for the patient to get out of bed. The sciatic portion of the syndrome with elements of numbness, weakness, severe leg pain to the foot or ankle, and burning or tingling parasthesias may not develop immediately, although this can occur. Rather, the sciatica often evolves gradually over the next several days or even weeks. Sometimes the lumbar portion of the syndrome can disappear with the pain being no more proximal than the buttocks.

The physical examination

The physical presentation of the lumbar spine is, as described in Chap. 4, with limitation of lumbar motion, muscle spasm, localized tenderness, list, and an awkward slow gait (in those patients with the complete syndrome). Movements are usually well controlled and careful.

There are three categories of tests in the physical examination that directly relate to the evaluation of the symptom of sciatica.

The first group of tests are designed to detect nerve root pressure, tension, or irritation of the sciatic nerve. The first and most important of these is the straight leg raising (SLR) test and its variant called Lasegue's sign (see Chap. 2). With the knee fully extended the involved leg is raised from the examining table. A positive SLR test requires reproduction of pain at an elevation of less than 60°. The production of lower back pain is not a positive

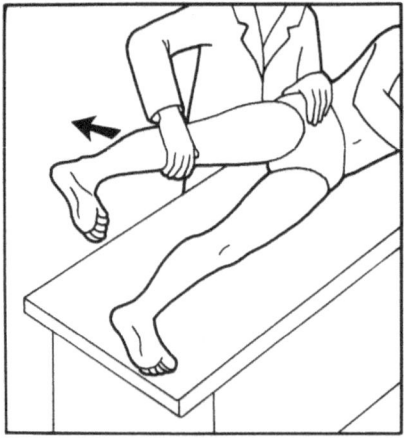

Fig. 1. The femoral stretch test

test of sciatica. The contralateral leg raising test (or "well leg raising test") is the same as the straight leg raising test but is positive when pain is produced in the opposite (affected) leg. A positive SLR is the single most important sign of nerve root pressure produced by a disc herniation while the contralateral leg raising test (when present) is nearly pathognomonic of disc herniation. It does not, however, indicate which root is affected. The femoral stretch test (the reverse of the straight leg raising test) (Fig. 1) is designed to place tension on the nerve roots above L4. Tenderness on direct pressure on the sciatic nerve in the sciatic notch indicates that the nerve is irritated but not why it is irritated.

The second group of tests is designed to detect which nerve root or roots is affected. The three most common roots to be involved are L4, L5, and S1. Spangfort (1972) summarized 49 publications with a total of 15,235 operations and found that in 47% the L5-S1 level was addressed, in 50% the L4-L5 level, and in 3% higher levels. Age influences the level at which the herniation is most frequently found (Fig. 2a). Thus below age 45 L5-S1 herniations dominate, while L4-L5 herniations dominate thereafter (Fig. 2b). Higher level herniations become more frequent with advancing age (Fig. 3). The L4 root dysfunction is indicated by a diminished patellar tendon reflex; altered sensation in the area immediately medial to the patella and down the anterior leg to the ankle and dorsal medial foot; and tibialis anterior weakness (see Chap. 2). L5 nerve root dysfunction is indicated by a sensory deficit on the anterior leg, dorsum of the foot and first web space; there is no reflex abnormality when the L5 root is involved; extensor hallucis longus weakness is specific for this root (see Chap. 2). The S1 root innervates the posterior thigh and calf muscles and, therefore, weakness in attempted toe walking is indicative of S1 root injury; S1 sensory dermatome is the lateral calf and lateral foot; the S1 reflex is the achilles tendon reflex (see

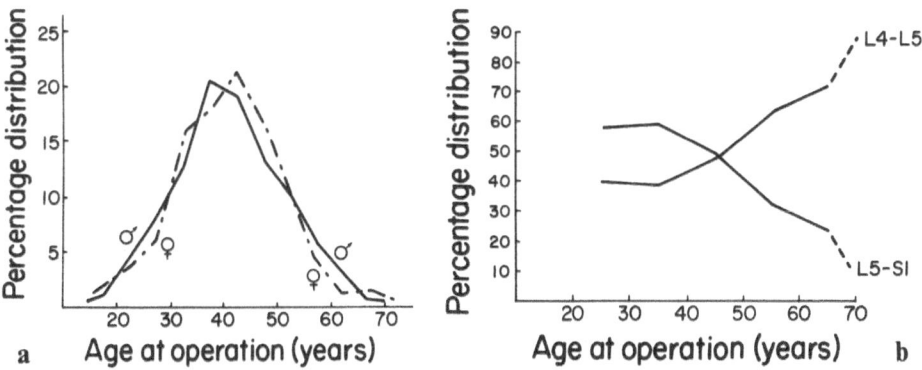

Fig. 2a, b. Percent distribution of disc hernia operations at L4-5 and L5-S1 levels as a function of age at operation. (Adapted from Spangfort, 1972)

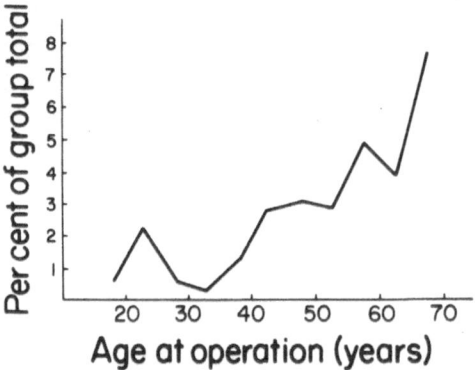

Fig. 3. Higher level herniations (above L4-5) become more common with advanced age. (Adapted from Spangfort, 1972)

Chap. 2). No specific reflex changes are present for lumbar nerves above L4 or below S1. Involvement of these nerve roots are uncommon, however. The L1, 2, 3 nerve roots innervate the anterior thigh and iliopsoas and quadriceps muscles while those below S1 innervate the plantar foot muscles, some of the posterior thigh and calf muscles, and the rectal and bladder muscles.

The third group are those tests which are designed to exclude intrathecal lesions involving the spinal cord or cauda equina. The first of these is the Milgrim test (Fig. 4). The Milgrim test requires that the patient holds both feet off of the examination table for thirty seconds. If this is possible, it is quite unlikely that the patient has an intrathecal lesion, but inability to perform the test yields no valuable new information. This test is not possible in the very acutely affected individual because of pain, but is useful in the subacute or chronic patient with sciatica. Several tests designed to raise the intrathecal

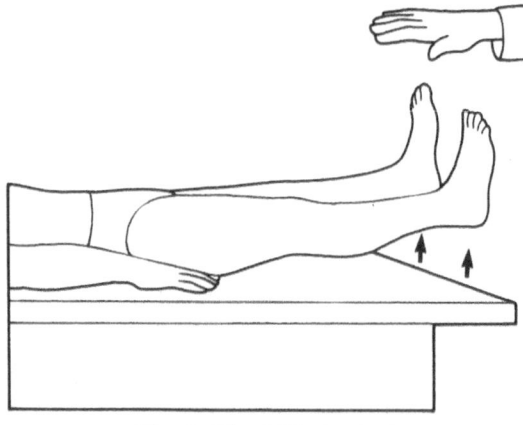

Fig. 4. The Milgrim test

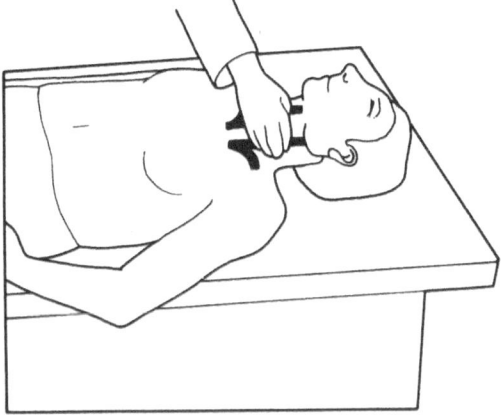

Fig. 5. Naffziger's test

pressure and thus detect lesions of the cord or cauda equina are available and require less strenuous muscular effort than the Milgrim test. Naffziger's test produces a similar result without patient effort. This test (Fig. 5) produces increased spinal fluid pressure by compression of the jugular veins. The Valsalva sign and Lhermitte's sign are intermediate in their requirement of patient effort. The Valsalva sign requires that the patient holds his breath and bears down as when initiating a bowel movement. The test is positive when pain is produced in the back or legs indicating either an intrathecal lesion or pressure on the thecal sac from without. Lhermitte's sign is positive when active neck flexion produces descending parathesias in the arms and legs indicating proximal spinal cord pathology. The Brudzinski sign (Fig. 6) pro-

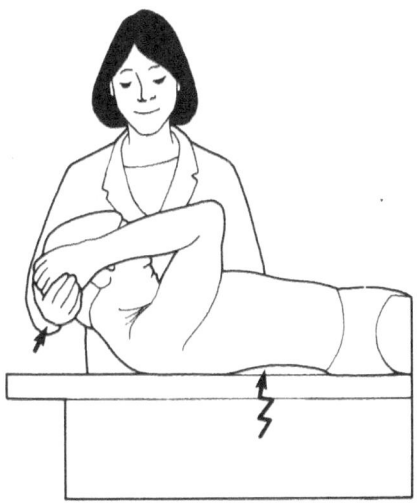

Fig. 6. Brudzinski's sign

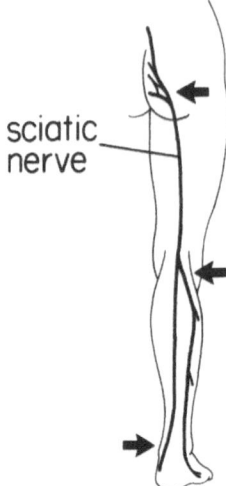

Fig. 7. Sites of distal nerve entrapment

duces back pain and spontaneous hip and knee flexion on attempted neck flexion. This indicates inflammatory exudate about the lumbar roots.

Babinski's sign is positive when the toes fan and extend on gentle stroking of the sole of the foot. A positive Babinski sign indicates an upper motor neuron lesion and should direct attention away from the lumbar spine to the central nervous system.

There are no specific tests on physical examination which are capable of detecting the unusual instance of nerve involvement below the level of the lumbar spine except the Tinell sign at the point of injury (Tinell's sign is the production of parasthesias by percussion of the nerve). This test may detect the site of nerve injury masquerading as sciatica at the knee, ankle, or foot (Fig. 7). It is not valuable for intrapelvic lesions or buttock lesions. Lesions of the nerves distal to the lumbar spine may paradoxically produce proximal symptoms and thus be doubly difficult to localize.

Pathologic correlates

Details of the pathologic changes in the lumbar intervertebral disc leading to the dramatic development of discal hernia has been presented in Chap. 1. Herniation of normal discs can be produced in the laboratory but only under rather extreme conditions of overload in flexion. Clinical disc hernias mainly occur in discs that have been previously weakened by the degenerative process (Fig. 8). A normal disc can herniate following severe trauma such as a fall from a height but even then bony injury is more likely.

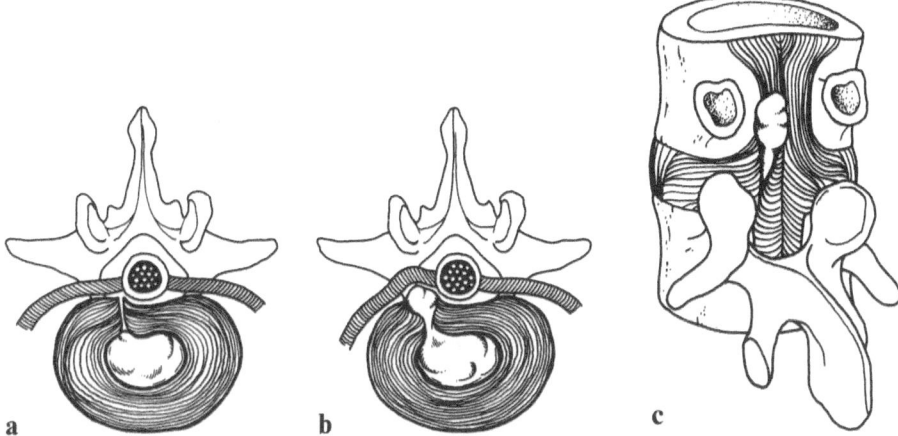

Fig. 8. a Annular tear; **b** disc protrusion through torn annulus; **c** extruded disc fragment migrating proximally

Investigations

Myelography, CT scanning, and MRI scanning all have a place in the diagnosis of the various causes of sciatica (see Chap. 2). Myelography is sensitive for central and posterolateral disc hernias above L5-S1 levels but may miss lateral herniations (Fig. 9) and herniations at L5-S1 if there is a wide anterior epidural space. Myelography is the most sensitive test for intra-thecal pathology, but MRI scans are proving sensitive in this respect also. CT is the best screening test for disc hernias and can be the only diagnostic test needed when the findings are unequivocal and correspond to the clinical syndrome. Post-

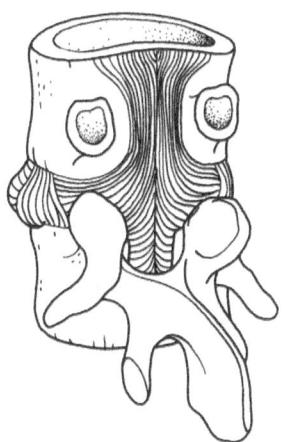

Fig. 9. Far lateral disc herniation

myelographic CT scans are quite helpful complements to specifically deline-
ate lesions, and detect more lateral herniations. There is little or no place for
discography except possibly the combination of discography and CT scanning for far lateral discal hernias. Lumbosacral and pelvic X-ray studies are
always appropriate, and should preceed the above tests. Bone scans are rarely
indicated but do have a place in selected cases of patients with sciatica (see
Chap. 2).

Conservative treatment

Bed rest for a few days and analgesic and antiinflammatory medications are
appropriate for up to six weeks if there is no progression of neurologic signs
or any severe neurologic sign such as in a cauda equina syndrome (Chap. 8).
It is almost always correct to wait six weeks before abandoning conservative
(non-operative) therapy. It is most important to appreciate that many patients with disc hernias are able to live and function normally after a period
of normal non-operative care. In ninety percent, patients with sciatica recover in ninety days. Further, patients treated conservatively are indistinguishable from those treated operatively at five, ten, and fifteen year follow-up
(Weber, 1983).

The patient with acute sciatica, when seen by the physician should, initially, be made comfortable and as relaxed as possible so that an adequate
history and physical examination can be done. When these are completed
plain lumbosacral spine radiographs should be taken and reviewed. If well
localized lumbar pain is not present, an AP pelvis radiograph may also be
required.

Almost all patients can be treated at home with a few days of modified
bed rest which would permit arising for the toilet, bath, and meals. Sitting is
to be strictly avoided. A posture with hip and knees flexed (assisted by pillow
or bolster) should be recommended. Narcotic pain medicine may be necessary for a few days but must not be prolonged. Non-steroidal antiinflammatory medication is quite helpful and is the cornerstone of the initial medical
treatment. A short course of methyl prednisolone (0.5 mg/kg/day) for 3 or 4
days can dramatically improve the symptoms. This treatment should be
avoided in patients with diabetes, ulcers, or an infectious process. Patients
with sciatica may require longer periods of rest than those with acute low
back pain alone, and the duration of the illness is often much longer than
when low back pain alone is present. Fifty percent of patients are better in
1 month and ninety percent are better in ninety days (Hakelius, 1970). Of ten
percent of patients with continued symptoms of sciatica (after ninety days)
only about one half to one fifth will require operative treatment.

Weber (1983), in a prospective study, has shown that only about one fifth of patients, randomized into a conservative therapy group, were unable to tolerate the continued symptoms and required surgery.

Surgical treatment

Surgical excision of the disc hernia remains the primary treatment in those cases that are very severe or do not respond to conservative care within six weeks.

Surgical removal of a herniated intervertebral disc, in a patient with definite findings on physical examination, definite radiographic confirmation with CT or myelography, and no secondary gain can be expected to yield ninety percent good results (Hirsch, 1963). The result of surgery is clearly related to the finding at operation. When dividing his material into complete herniations (extruded disc fragments), incomplete herniations (well defined circumscribed lesions clearly protruding beyond anatomic limits), and bulging discs (generalized bulges of disc protruding beyond normal anatomic limits), and negative explorations, Spangfort (1972) found that complete relief can almost be expected with complete and incomplete herniations, but that patients with bulges have only a 63 % complete relief and those with no herniation a 37 % relief (Fig. 10). Results in his study tended to be less good with advancing age. In our opinion, only patients with clear cut findings of disc hernias on structural examinations and appropriate clinical signs and symptoms should be operated on. Weber (1978) has shown that the surgery is more effective if done earlier than twelve weeks, and that surgery leads to a more rapid recovery than conservative treatment.

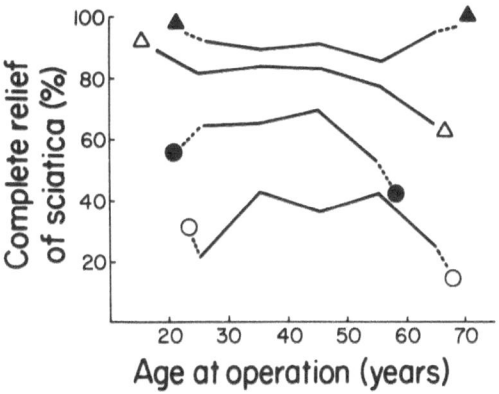

Fig. 10. Results of disc surgery depends on the finding. ▲ Complete herniation, △ incomplete herniation, ● bulging disc, ○ no herniation. (Adapted from Spangfort, 1972)

Conversely, patients with secondary gain or psychologic disturbance are more likely to have an unsatisfactory outcome following surgery (McNeill et al., 1987).

Chemonucleolysis is an alternative treatment which is of value in instances in which the disc hernia is not extruded or not extremely large (Fraser, 1984; McCulloch, 1980; Postacchini et al., 1987). The results on ten year follow up compare favorably with surgical treatment (Weinstein et al., 1986). However, this treatment is not without risk and must not be considered to be a "lesser treatment" than surgical disc removal.

Epidural steroids have been controversial. Very short term follow-up of twenty-four hours in a random study (Cuckler et al., 1985) revealed no improvement over saline. However, other studies (Dilke et al., 1973; Kahanovitz, 1986) have shown significant short term improvement, in 60% of patient with sciatica. We experienced no improvement in patients with discal herniations but reasonable improvement, for the short term, in patients with spinal stenosis and bony nerve root entrapment. Frymoyer (1988) also suggests the use of epidural steroid injections in some patients.

Percutaneous suction discectomy has recently been introduced but has not yet found its appropriate place (if any) in the treatment of disc hernia.

7 The patient with severe unremitting lower back pain

Introduction

In each of the chapters in this book a syndrome has been described which should lead the physician to a progressively more narrow choice of diagnoses. The opposite is true with the uncommon and often perplexing patient with severe unremitting lower back pain. Patients with many different diseases may, at some point in the course of the illness, complain of constant pain in the back. These patients form a subset of several of the different low back pain syndromes. The complaint can also be present in a group of vascular causes of lower back pain some of which are well known and some of which are gradually becoming elucidated. Patients with severe unremitting low back pain can be divided into acute, subacute and chronic groups based on presentation of symptoms (Table 1).

Table 1. Differential diagnostic categories of back pain patients presenting with severe unremitting low back pain

Acute	Subacute	Chronic	Uncommon
Vascular	Tumor	Vascular	Congenital
Trauma	Infection	Inflammatory	
Infection	Degenerative	Degenerative	
Tumor	Inflammatory	Metabolic	
Degenerative		Infection	
Psychiatric		Developmental	
		Psychiatric	
		Post-traumatic	
		Tumor	

Acute unremitting low back pain

Amongst patients with lower back pain the potential for life threatening or disabling illness is greatest in the group of patients with acute, severe, and unremitting, lower back pain. Each of these patients, therefore, requires very careful analysis and rapid decision making.

Abdominal aortic aneurysm

The rupture of an abdominal aortic aneurysm is a surgical emergency which requires prompt diagnosis and treatment in order to save the patient (Table 2). Typically this patient is an elderly individual with a previous history of hypertension. The presentation is often dramatic with severe sharp abdominal or lower back pain often brought on by lifting or straining. Sciatica and lower extremity nerve dysfunction is common. The patient may show extreme anxiety and thrash about. He may become ashen, confused, and diaphoretic with increasing hypotension progressing to shock. Dissection of the aneurysm can lead to paraplegia due to obstruction of the arterial supply to the spinal cord. The physical examination will reveal a pulsatile, tender, abdominal swelling often with an associated bruit. Pulses may be absent in the legs. Immediate surgical treatment is required.

Table 2. Symptoms and signs of ruptured aortic aneurysm

History	Physical
Hypertension	Tender, pulsatile swelling
Elderly	Hypotension/shock
Sudden onset	Pulseless legs
Sharp constant pain	Paraplegia rarely

Trauma

Trauma to the spine can obviously produce severe unremitting lower back pain. The nature of the illness will seldom be missed as the history and circumstances of the patient's arrival should, in most instances, make the probable diagnosis obvious. The problem with most spinal trauma patients is proper sequential assessment without adding to the injury. The patient must be moved from the scene of the injury without flexing or twisting the spine. He must be transported on a rigid surface. The first concerns with trauma patients are the provision of an airway and hemodynamic stability. These goals must be achieved before attention is specifically directed to the spine problem. However, they must not be achieved at the expense of the spinal alignment, stability or damage to neural tissue. Spinal fractures are sometimes overlooked because of associated injuries to other parts of the body. This is particularly dangerous since emergency surgery is often necessary in these multiply injured patients. Special care of the spine to prevent additional injury is particularly important in the defenseless anesthetized patient.

Infection

Infections may produce severe and unremitting lower back pain with an acute onset (see Chap. 15). Acute pyogenic osteomyelitis of the spine is today, most often, a disease of adults. It commonly follows GU or GYN manipulation and may be associated with fever, chills, and malaise. Pain is sometimes localized to the buttocks, groin, or abdomen in addition to the lower back. The pain is typically unrelieved by rest. Radicular symptoms may be present.

Discitis

Discitis is a primary disease of children and an iatrogenic disease of adults (Tables 3 and 4). Direct seeding of a disc space via the hematogenous route can occur only when blood vessels enter the space. This condition is met in children but not in adults unless pathologic neovascularization has taken place. In both children and adults the back pain may have a rather acute onset and be quite severe and constant. In very young children the symptoms may include refusal to walk, abdominal pain and back pain. In both children and adults the physical findings are localized back tenderness with spasm. Fever and other generalized findings may be absent (see Chap. 15).

Table 3. Symptoms and signs of discitis in childhood

History	Signs
Irritable	Local tenderness
Refusal to walk	Some with fever
Abdominal pain	Limitation of motions with guarding
"Hip" pain	
Constant pain	

Table 4. Symptoms and signs of discitis in adults

History	Signs
Post injection	Severe spasm
Post surgical	Severe limitation of motion
Acute or insidious onset	Flat back
Severe back pain	Neurologic usually negative
Constant pain	

Tumor

Both primary and metastatic tumors involving the bone or epidural space can present with a rather sudden onset of lower back pain with or without radicular complaints. Most often the acute onset of severe unremitting lower back pain in a tumor patient is due to a pathologic fracture; although, epidural extension with involvement of neural elements may also result in severe localized pain (see Chap. 14).

Acute discal hernia

From a pathologic point of view, acute discal hernia is not a primary trauma related process. Nonetheless, patients often describe an "injury" which is usually trivial. As discussed in Chap. 6, disc hernias usually do not produce severe unremitting pain. Rather pain is usually related to posture and activity. Massive disc herniation can produce severe and unremitting lower back pain, however. This situation is not trivial and can result in a cauda equina syndrome (see Chap. 8) with permanent deficit in sensation of the lower extremities, bladder dysfunction and sexual dysfunction (Table 5). In patients with severe unremitting lower back pain and urinary retention myelography is often an urgent consideration. Rarely, an intrathecal tumor may have a similar presentation and again myelography is required.

Table 5. Cauda equina syndrome*

History	Signs
Previous lower back pain	Saddle anesthesia
Bilateral sciatica	Enlarged bladder
Inability to void	Numbness of the soles of the feet
Severe lower back pain	Straight leg raising positive bilaterally
Perineal pain	Absent anal "wink"
Parasthesias	

* Unilateral sciatica is possible

Subacute unremitting low back pain

The above mentioned conditions may also have a subacute presentation. The group of *(seronegative) inflammatory arthritides* of the spine are more likely to have a subacute presentation (see Chap. 16). Young males presenting with moderate lower back pain which is almost always present but worse in the morning and worse after heavy activity but which is partially relieved by moderate activity should be evaluated for ankylosing spondylitis.

Other suggestive clues to the possible diagnosis of inflammatory arthritis of the spine are the association of low back pain to (1) inflammatory bowel disease; (2) psoriasis; (3) inflammatory eye symptoms; and (4) previous gastrointestinal or urinary tract infections.

Chronic unremitting low back pain

Chronic low back pain may be caused by many categories of disease (Table 1). However, for the pain to be severe, chronic and unremitting is quite unusual (Chap. 10). In most chronic pain conditions, there are significant periods of respite from the pain. The pain from osteoporosis, degenerative disease, spondylolisthesis (developmental), immunologic and post traumatic spinal conditions tends to be intermittent. In some instances pain is present on a daily basis and in other instances the period between episodes of pain is much longer. *Tumors* and *untreated chronic infections* are the most common exceptions to this general rule.

Intrathecal adhesions (arachnoiditis) from trauma, infection, surgical treatment, and myelography can result in severe low back pain, too. This pain can be unremitting but usually does respond to rest. The reason for pain in patients with intrathecal adhesions is believed to be decreased microcirculation of the nerve roots and is thus a "vascular" cause of chronic unremitting lower back pain.

Functional unremitting low back pain

Psychiatric or *psychological* causes of low back pain are not uncommon and are often described as constant (see Chap. 13) (Table 6).

Table 6. Functional pain complaint

History	Physical
Secondary gain	Cutaneous tenderness
Diffuse pain	Distraction positive
Nonanatomic pain	Nonanatomic sensory or motor
Sleep disturbance	"Academy Award"
"La belle indifference"	
In appropriate use of emergency services	
Excessive demands	

There are many subgroups of psychiatric illness with pain complaint including malingering. A careful history should always be directed toward finding symptoms of depression and sources of secondary gain. Each patient examination should include Waddell's non-organic physical signs (Chap. 2).

Summary

Unremitting severe low back pain is uncommon. When occurring acutely severe disease should be suspected and the diagnostic workup should be thorough and urgent. Chronic or subacute unremitting low back pain is even more rare. Infections and inflammatory conditions must be excluded. Treatment in these patients is specific to the underlying cause. In our opinion, these patients should be cared for by someone specialized in low back disorders.

8 The patient with lower back pain, sciatica, and inability to void

Introduction

The constellation of signs and symptoms listed in Group D of Table 1 are known collectively as the "cauda equina syndrome". The distinguishing feature of this syndrome is the involvement of the sacral roots below the S-1 level. These symptoms distinguish the cauda equina syndrome from acute benign lower back pain (Group A), acute lower back pain with radicular symptoms (Group C) and the lower back pain which is not primarily spinal in origin (Group B). In the early reports on disc operations this, most severe of the disc hernia syndromes, was represented by a disproportionate number

Table 1. Lower lumbar – upper sacral pain

A Acute – benign	*B* Chronic – visceral
Sudden onset	Gradual onset
Relieved by rest	Un-relieved by rest
Aggravated by motion	Not aggravated by motion
Radiation no lower than thigh	Upper lumbar pain
Local spinal tenderness	Flank pain
Flat back	Hematuria/dysuria
Fetal position = comfort	Positive "Murphy punch"
Possible list	Abdominal tenderness
"Spasm"	Abdominal mass
Limitation of spinal motion	Rectal pain/bleeding
Non-radicular	Previous malignancy
Age usually under 40	Age greater than 50
C Acute – radicular	*D* Acute – cauda equina syndrome
As in *A* group	As in *A* or *C* group
Radiation below the knee	With perineal numbness
Associated parathesias	With urinary retention
Associated weakness	With incontinence
Positive stretch test	With bilateral sciatica
Reflex change	Loss of rectal tone
Sciatic notch tenderness	Paraparesis

of cases. Seven of Mixter and Barr's original cases had a variation of this syndrome. Large recent studies (Spangfort, 1972; Raaf, 1959) indicate that the actual incidence of cauda equina syndrome in patients with disc herniation is low; closer to two percent overall. It is important to recognize that disc herniation is not the only cause of cauda equina syndrome; but, it is by far the most common. Other causes of sacral root neural compression are tumors and infections.

Typical history

There are two general groups of patients with cauda equina syndrome (Shephard, 1959). In the first group, the syndrome develops slowly over a period of months or years; and, in the second group, some or all of the features of the syndrome develop suddenly within one to seven days. We shall refer to the first, and smaller, group as "chronic cauda equina syndrome" and the second group as "acute cauda equina syndrome". This distinction has clinical relevance since the prognosis differs between the groups.

Chronic cauda equina syndrome

The chronic cauda equina patient presents with symptoms of urinary incontinence, hesitancy or urgency of long duration and of gradually increasing severity. The patients may complain of perianal or perineal pain. The patients may also suffer from pain in the legs with walking. The leg pains, when present, are quite similar to those of vascular insufficiency but signs of arterial disease are absent. These pains are typically relieved by sitting or even leaning forward at the waist (pseudo-claudication). In addition to their urinary problems, the patients may also describe some degree of fecal incontinence. Patients in the chronic group are usually older than fifty, while patients in the acute group have a mean age of about forty years. The chronic patients give no recent history of injury to the lower back, but symptoms of sciatica and back ache may have been present for many years.

Acute cauda equina syndrome

The acute group may present itself in three different patterns: (I) A sudden onset of cauda equina syndrome without previous symptoms; (II) An onset of cauda equina syndrome in a patient who has had previous episodes of lower back pains and sciatica; (III) The patient with bilateral sciatica (rarely with unilateral sciatica) and low back pain who goes on to develop cauda equina syndrome. [Patterns I, II, and III are described by Tandon and Sankaran (1967), the variation with unilateral sciatica is extensively described by Floman et al. (1980)] (Table 2).

Table 2. Acute cauda equina syndrome

I	Sudden onset
	No previous symptoms
II	Sudden onset
	Previous lower back pain and sciatica
III	Presenting with sciatica with later development of cauda equina syndrome

In Group I of acute patients, the primary complaint can be low back and perianal pain with bilateral sciatica being secondary or even occasionally absent. Severe, incapacitating low back pain is a constant feature as is urinary retention. The distribution of the sciatica is usually buttocks, posterior thigh and leg, and includes the sole of the foot. There is often a history of overload usually a lifting "accident".

Group II is distinguished from Group I by a history of previous attacks of low back pain with sciatica which have responded to conservative care. However, the current episode is more severe than the previous attacks and is associated with urinary retention.

Group III patients present with bilateral sciatica (rarely with unilateral sciatica) and then go on to develop the additional symptoms of cauda equina syndrome. When the symptoms are unilateral and typical of the more benign version of discal hernia the development of urinary retention may be thought to be due to bed rest, pain or analgesics used as treatment for back pain and sciatica; and, in fact, most instances of urinary retention are due to inhibition due to unaccustomed bed rest, pain and narcotic medication. Because of the frequent occurrence of benign urinary retention in these circumstances and because of their rarity, Group III patients always come as a great surprise to the clinician responsible for their care. Vigilance in the care of these patients is essential as the syndrome may be evolving at the time of initial contact, but the potential for the development of a severe illness may not be appreciated. This is especially true since the recommended care for low back pain with or without sciatica consists of bed rest and pain relieving medication, a treatment that differs radically from that of a cauda equina syndrome. Further, one should note that the classical description of a cauda equina syndrome usually ignores the fact that the presentation may be unilateral rather than bilateral sciatica.

Physical examination

The sine qua non of the cauda equina syndrome is urinary retention; and, therefore, the findings of bladder distention with palpable and percussable

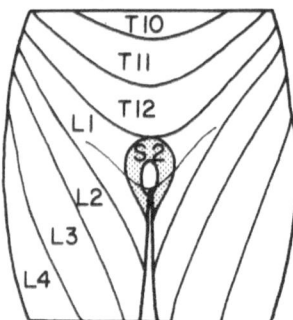 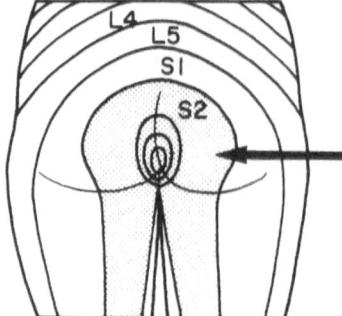

Fig. 1. Sensory distribution of sacral nerves

bladder enlargement associated with lower abdominal tenderness is always present. The findings of wide-spread numbness in the perineum, buttock, posterior thighs, posterior calves, and soles of the feet is typical of the full blown syndrome (Fig. 1). However, the findings in a lower limb can be unilateral; and, yet, severe bladder involvement may be present. Anal wink may be absent and anal sphincter tone may be diminished. The straight leg raising test is almost always positive. The finding of weakness in the limbs is variable, as are reflex abnormalities. Flattening of the normal lumbar lordosis, diminished lumbar range of motion, with spasm and list are also common. The gait is antalgic and strength as tested by heel and toe walking is frequently abnormal.

Pathological correlates

In the chronic variation of the cauda equina syndrome the sacral nerve root compression develops slowly. Most often this is due to gradual loss of volume of the lumbar spinal canal as a function of lumbar spondylosis (spinal stenosis) (Chap. 9). There may be associated discal annular bulging due to loss of the nuclear material and secondary loss of disc height. The thecal sac thus becomes compressed on all four sides; laterally, by the enlarging degenerative facets; anteriorly, by the bulging annulus; and, posteriorly, by the lamina of the lower level sliding under the lamina of the adjacent level with the ligamentum flavum folding under it, thus adding to the posterior component of the stenosis. This is the process as it develops in the elderly patient. Occasionally, a chronic cauda equina syndrome may develop in a younger patient, however. In this instance, the stenosis is of the congenital variety and decompensation of the nervous structures is the result of central and gradual discal herniation. Rarely is the chronic variety of cauda equina syndrome the result of a slowly expanding intrathecal lesion such as a neurolemmoma.

Acute cauda equina syndrome is almost always the result of an acute disc hernia (Tay and Chacha, 1979). The herniation is most often at one of the two lower lumbar segments (L4–5 and L5-S1); but, proportionately more of the upper lumbar herniations produce cauda equina syndrome than do lower herniations. In other words, upper lumbar herniations are responsible for a greater fraction of the total number of cauda equina compressions than their overall incidence would suggest, and a very high proportion of the intrathecal herniations (Peyser and Harari, 1977) produce cauda equina syndrome (Fig. 2). Fortunately, intrathecal herniations are very rare (1 to 2 per 1000 herniations). Even massive disc herniations (Fig. 3) may not produce cauda equina syndrome, but the combination of a large herniation and a small spinal canal makes its development more probable. It is this unfortunate combination of factors that most often leads to iatrogenic cauda equina syndrome. The attempted removal of a large central disc herniation, through the usual interlaminar approach, with concomitant swelling or haematoma in the closed space produced by the retained lamina, may produce sufficient pressure to injure the intrathecal nerve roots.

It is common for male patients with cauda equina syndrome to have some significant sexual dysfunction. The associated motor paralysis tends to recover in part after adequate decompression. However, bladder dysfunction may not recover well and residual changes may be evident years later. This is less likely when the original symptoms are unilateral. It is thought that this is due to the sensory portion of the neural injury having been post ganglionic and not subject to recovery; and, thus, the bladder atonia is due, at least in part, to loss of the normal bladder reflex arc. Whereas, the unilaterally involved patients have retained a portion of the sensory mechanism; and, therefore, have a somewhat better prognosis for recovery of bladder function. This agrees with the observation that bladder function may be retained in patients who have undergone hemi-sacrectomy for tumors.

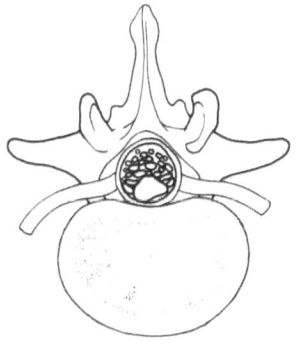

Fig. 2. Intrathecal disc hernia

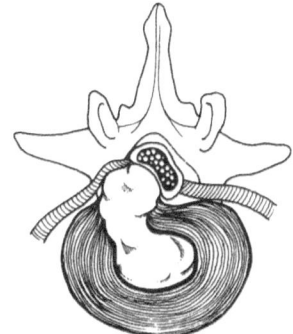

Fig. 3. Massive disc hernia

Investigations

In patients presenting with the chronic variety of cauda equina syndrome there is no immediate urgency in the need for treatment and so the workup can be deliberate and complete. This should include complete urologic studies including IVP, urine cultures, kidney function testing, and obtaining a cystometrogram. Complete lumbosacral spine studies should be done including radiographs and myelography. In some instances, these might be supplemented with CT and MRI studies.

In the patient with the acute variety of cauda equina syndrome there is urgency in the treatment which is a surgical decompression; and, therefore, the studies should be limited to those which allow proper surgical planning. These necessary studies are lumbar spine radiographs and myelography. Sometimes MRI can replace myelography. In patients where it is unclear whether a bladder paralysis is neurogenic or due to pain, cystometry can be helpful. These patients will not have perianal anesthesia.

Treatment

In both the acute and chronic varieties of the cauda equina syndrome the only treatment is complete decompression of the involved neural elements. Where massive disc herniation is the cause of the neural compression hemilaminectomy and discectomy has been selected as the treatment of choice in one series (Aho et al., 1969). However, almost all surgeons would elect a total laminectomy (and discectomy when appropriate) for their patients with cauda equina syndrome, and we certainly subscribe to this.

In the acute cauda equina syndrome the procedure should be performed as a medical emergency. However, a proper level diagnosis must precede any procedure as well as an exclusion of the very rare tumor cause of this syndrome.

Results

Surgical decompression is much more likely to result in complete, or nearly complete, resolution of symptoms in patients with the chronic cauda equina syndrome than in patients with the acute variety. Most authors in the past have urged that the patients with acute cauda equina syndrome be treated the same day as it occurs with surgical decompression. This degree of urgency is supported by the available clinical evidence to some extent. Aho et al. (1969) demonstrated that the results of surgical decompression on recovery of bladder function became significantly less good if the delay in treatment was greater than two days. Other investigators (Shephard, 1959) recommend early decompression on the theoretical basis that one cannot tell which neural injuries are partial and which are complete on clinical grounds. Although the average duration of symptoms in most published series has been far greater than two days without significant alteration in the results; we must recommend that the surgery be performed within the shortest time commensurate with safe handling of the patient and accurate localization of the lesion. This last aspect is critical, however, and surgery should never be performed without adequate localization of the lesion.

9 The patient with lower back pain and leg pain with walking

Introduction

The concept of "spinal stenosis" began to evolve in the 1940s in Europe. Verbiest (1954) should be credited with starting the development of the modern concept of this most complex of the many lower back pain syndromes. The word "stenosis", in this context, implies a narrowing of the spinal canal, not caused by a disc herniation alone. This narrowing may involve the central canal and/or the exit canals for the individual nerve roots.

History

More variation exists in the presenting complaints in this group of patients than in any other of the syndromes producing low back pain (Table 1). However, there are three recognizable subsyndromes of "spinal stenosis". These are: pseudo claudication; radicular (sciatica) (Chap. 6); chronic cauda equina syndrome (Chap. 8). Pseudo claudication is the unique syndrome singling out the concept of spinal stenosis, but individual patients may present with almost any conceivable combination of these complaints. Further-

Table 1. Characteristics of the patient with lower back pain and leg pain when walking

Patient is more often older then 50 years
Morning pain and stiffness
Sitting relieves the pain
Leaning forward relieves the pain
Extension aggravates the pain
Leg symptoms often bilateral
Leg pain more common than either weakness or parasthesias
Walking aggravates or produces the leg symptoms
Gradual onset of sphincter disturbance – slow and subtle
Symptoms of long duration and gradually increasing

more, an individual patient may have any one or several of these syndromes at different times during the course of the illness.

Often, the patients have had some complaints of low back pain for several years before seeking medical attention. The most common complaint of these patients is that of back pain (Porter et al., 1980). This lower back pain may be typical of spondylosis with morning stiffness relieved by mild limbering exercises but aggravated by moderate walking; the "gelling phenomena" with stiffness following any period of rest may be present. The pain is mild or absent with sitting. Patients with pseudo claudication (spinal stenosis) and true claudication (arteriosclerotic peripheral vascular disease – ASPVD) (Table 2) both experience leg pain with walking which is relieved by rest. Both groups of patients are likely to be older than fifty years. Unfortunately, some patients may have both pseudo claudication and true claudication since both are relatively common. In the patient with pure pseudo claudication the posture while walking is one of flexed back (Fig. 1). Extension of the spine will provoke symptoms (Fig. 2) while flexion will relieve them. The patients may be able to walk only a few hundred meters but will be able to ride a bicycle for kilometers. Peripheral vascular changes are absent: pulses are present; skin color is normal; hair and nails are normal; skin temperature is normal; and signs of neuropathy are absent.

Riding a stationary bicycle for exercise will provoke symptoms in ASPVD (Dyck et al., 1977). Further, the disappearance of symptoms with rest is often more rapid in vascular claudication; not infrequently is there an element of remaining pain and discomfort in the SS patient. Walking can also provoke paresthesias and weakness in the patient with stenosis; who may also experience "drop attacks" or sudden tendency to fall while walking.

Parasthesias, weakness and numbness with sciatica are also common complaints in patients with spinal stenosis (Epstein et al., 1962). These are

Table 2. Signs and symptoms in patients with true claudication and pseudo-claudication

Pseudo-claudication	True claudication
Leg pain with walking	Leg pain with walking
Relieved by rest	Relieved by rest
Aggravated by lumbar extension	Not aggravated by lumbar extension
Relieved by spinal flexion	Not relieved by spinal flexion
Bicycle not provocative	Bicycle provocative
Peripheral pulses present	Peripheral pulses absent
Trophic changes absent	Trophic changes present
Peripheral neuropathy absent	Peripheral neuropathy may be present
Flexed posture with walking	Flexed posture absent

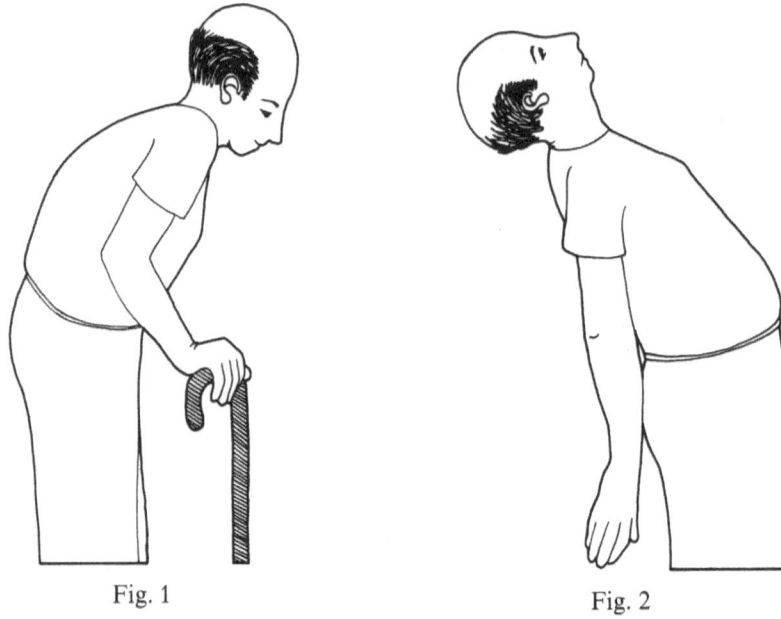

Fig. 1   Fig. 2

Fig. 1. Walking flexed in patient with spinal stenosis

Fig. 2. Extension aggravates symptoms in patient with spinal stenosis

often typical of an individual lumbar nerve root and are referred to as "radiculopathy" which is distinct from pseudo claudication (Chap. 6).

Approximately five percent of the patients will have groin, perianal, vulvar or testicular pain which may be associated with a chronic cauda equina syndrome (see Chap. 8).

Physical findings

The physical findings in SS are even less specific than is the patient's history. Examination of the back is often not revealing at all. The range of motion, although often reduced, is better than is found in patients with disc hernias, and acute low back pain and sciatica. In the elderly patient the degree of stiffness is compatible with their age; although, there is more often a structural deformity such as a rigid scoliosis or loss of lordosis. There is seldom any significant degree of local tenderness. Neurological signs such as weakness, numbness, reflex change or straight leg raising signs may be present only after exercise and disappear rapidly with rest. Unequivocal radicular findings are present only in a minority of cases. Straight leg raising and other nerve tension tests are usually negative.

Pathological correlates

The classification of spinal stenosis includes both an anatomic classification and an etiologic classification. The anatomic classification describes the portion or portions of the spinal canal which are narrowed. The central canal may be narrowed in either the anterior posterior dimension (sagittal plane) (Fig. 3) or the transverse dimension (coronal plane) (Fig. 4). This type of stenosis is referred to as *central stenosis*. Significant A-P diameter narrowing can occur on a hereditary basis. Narrowing to ten millimeters or less in this diameter represents "absolute spinal stenosis" (Rothman and Glenn, 1985), and narrowing between ten and fifteen mm is "relative stenosis" (Eisenstein, 1980) (Fig. 4). Stenosis secondary to congenital interpedicular narrowing is quite rare, but narrowing in the coronal plane due to medialized facets (trefoil

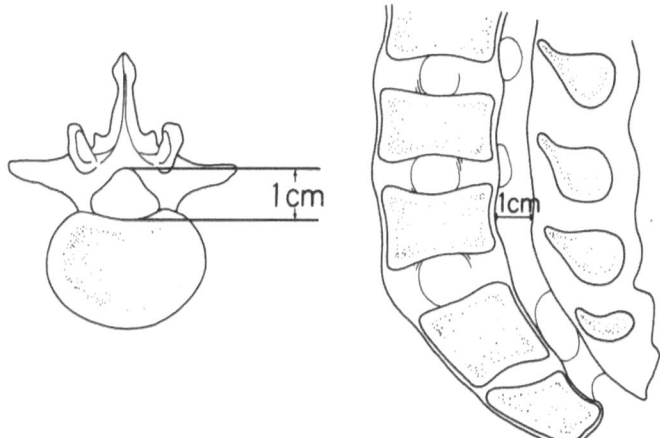

Fig. 3. Central canal measurements in spinal stenosis

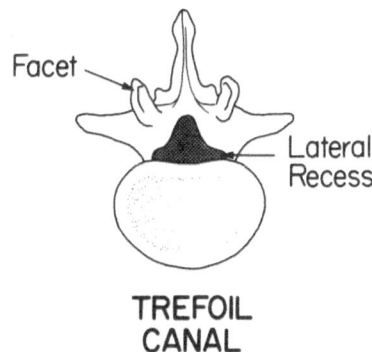

Fig. 4. Transverse canal narrowing and lateral recess stenosis in spinal stenosis

canal) is common (Eisenstein, 1980) (Fig. 4). Constriction of the thecal sac and its sensitive neural contents produces symptoms either by direct neural pressure or by constriction of the vaso nervorum or both.

The nerve root exits from the dural sac and then traverses three spinal zones (Fig. 5). Zone 1 is the so called "lateral recess" which is the area under the articular process and medial to the pedicle. Zone 2 is the portion of the nerve root canal which is immediately distal to the pedicle. Zone 3 is the area lateral to the pedicle. Nerve root entrapment occurs in any of these three zones, and is then referred to as *lateral stenosis*. In Zone 1 the constriction is due to enlargement of the facet and hypertrophic spurring secondary to spondylosis. As the nerve root crosses the disc at the beginning of Zone 1, a "hammer and anvil" effect may be produced by the bulging of the annulus secondary to disc degeneration under the root pushing it against the hypertrophic facet above (Fig. 6); or further along in Zone 1 osteophytes from the under surface of the facet may impinge upon the root. Constriction of the root in Zone 1 can have several causes. With loss of disc height secondary to spondylosis or disc resorption there may be a secondary subluxation of the facet joint with entrapment of the root between the superior facet of the inferior vertebra and the pedicle (Fig. 7). In this instance, the facet need not touch the root. The ligamentum flavum is pushed ahead of the advancing facet from the lower vertebra and obliterates the neuroforamen by filling it with extraneous soft tissue. In Zone 2 the root is close to the vertebral body and the adjacent pedicle, and it is secured in place by several small ligaments. In instances in which there is degenerative disc disease an enlarged "uncinate spur" or osteophyte from the vertebral margin can impinge upon the root at its most sensitive portion (the sensory ganglion). Asymmetric disc collapse with degenerative scoliosis can result in kinking of the root around the pedicle without actual neuroforamenal narrowing. Entrapment may occur in Zone 3 but is much less common than that occurring in the first two zones.

Both degenerative spondylolisthesis (Macnab, 1950) and spondylitic spondylolisthesis can produce spinal stenosis, but they do this by entirely

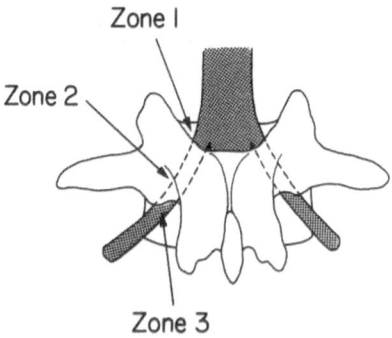

Fig. 5. Zones in lateral stenosis

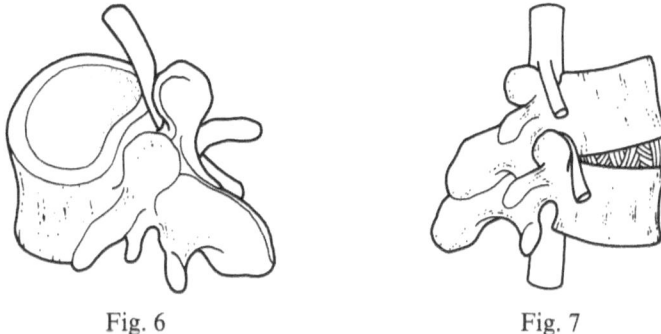

Fig. 6   Fig. 7

Fig. 6. Facet enlargement producing lateral stenosis and nerve root injury

Fig. 7. Disc narrowing producing neuroforamenal stenosis in extension

different mechanisms. In instances of spondylitic spondylolisthesis the area of stenosis is in Zone 2 of the nerve root canal. The posterior aspect of Zone 2 is formed normally by the pars interarticularis. This portion of the lamina has been disrupted in spondylitic spondylolisthesis with the formation of a fibrous pseudo-arthrosis and an "elephant foot" deformity of the detached posterior portion of the pedicle. This results in the formation of a markedly narrowed Zone 2 (Fig. 8). Thus, the nerve root when making its transit through this zone is liable to injury; but, fortunately, injury is not inevitable as this deformity is quite common without stenotic symptoms.

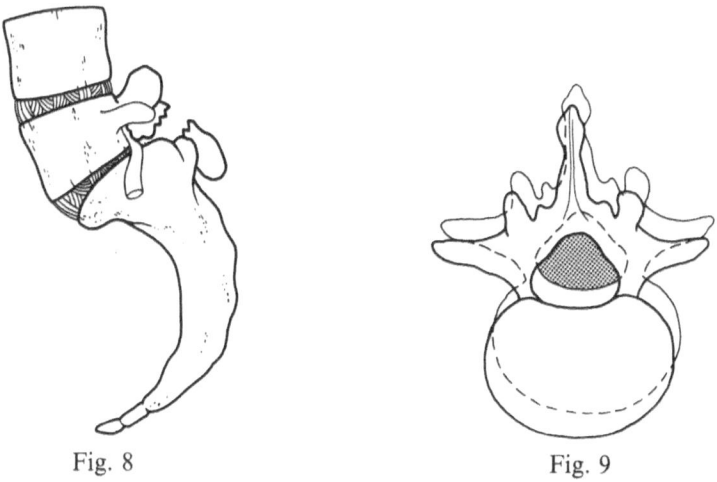

Fig. 8   Fig. 9

Fig. 8. Foramenal stenosis in isthmic spondylolisthesis

Fig. 9. Degenerative spondylolisthesis producing central stenosis

Degenerative spondylolisthesis produces a quite different form of spinal stenosis. In this instance, degeneration of the three joint complex (facets and disc) results in laxity of the annulus coupled with deformity of the facet cartilagenous surface resulting in forward slip of the proximal vertebra on its distal adjacent mate. Here the lamina of the slipping (proximal) vertebra remains rigidly attached to the pedicle and does not allow for compensatory enlargement of the AP diameter of the canal as occurs in spondylitic spondylolisthesis. Thus, a relatively small slip with an intact lamina produces a disproportionately large degree of central canal stenosis (Fig. 9).

As might be expected, the more likely clinical syndrome in patients with central stenosis and degenerative spondylolisthesis will be pseudo claudication. In a recent unpublished review of 92 of our patients, 73 percent of those with central stenosis or degenerative spondylolisthesis had bilateral leg pains with walking. In contradistinction in patients with lateral recess stenosis or neuroforamenal stenosis the predominant complaint was likely to be sciatica with pseudo claudication being secondary.

An etiologic classification of spinal stenosis is also of value as a compliment to the above anatomic classification, and is provided in Table 3 (Arnoldi et al., 1976).

Table 3. Classification of spinal stenosis. (From Arnoldi et al., 1976)

I.   Congenital – Developmental Stenosis
   a)   Idiopathic (hereditary)
   b)   Achondroplastic
II. Acquired Stenosis
   a)   Degenerative
   b)   Combined congenital and degenerative stenosis
   c)   Spondylolytic/Spondylolisthetic
   d)   Iatrogenic
      i)   Post laminectomy
      ii)   Post fusion
      iii) Post chemonucleolysis
   e)   Post traumatic
   f)   Metabolic
      i)   Paget's disease
      ii)   Fluorosis

The sequence of changes which lead to degenerative spinal stenosis have been summarized by Kirkaldy-Willis et al. (1978, 1984) (Fig. 10).

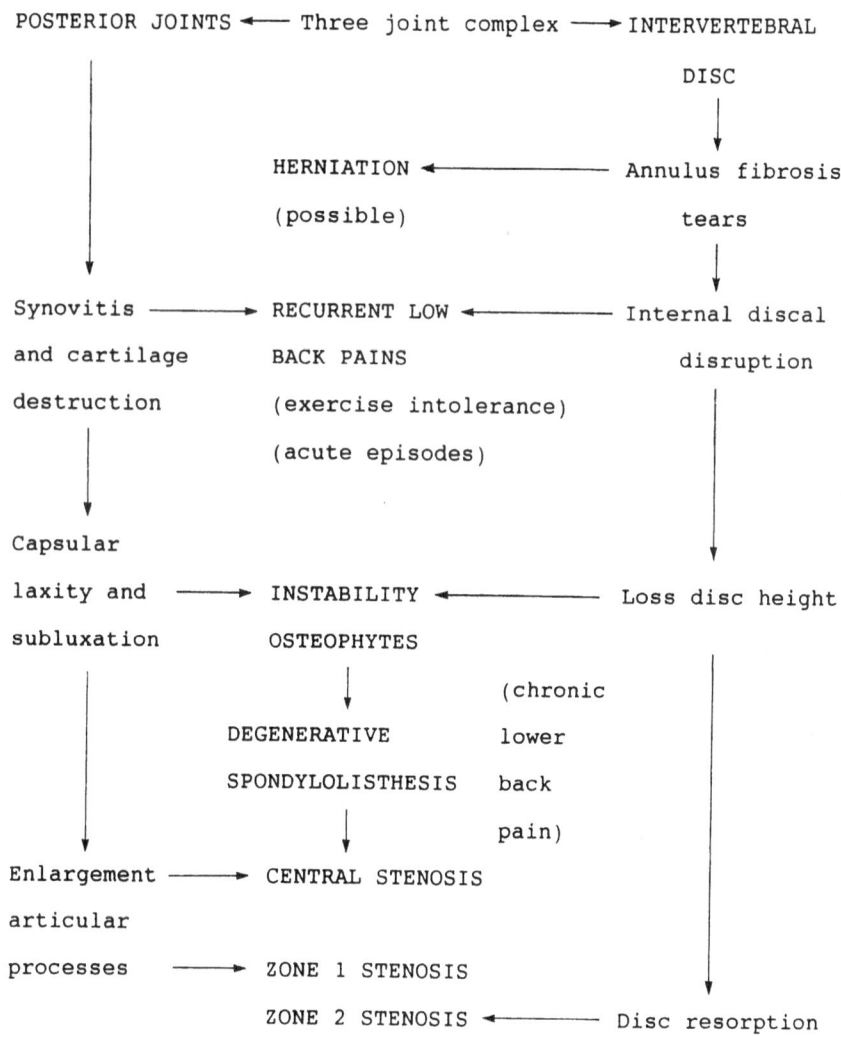

Fig. 10. Sequence of changes leading to degenerative spinal stenosis. (After Kirkaldy-Willis et al., 1978)

Investigations

Central stenosis on either a developmental or acquired basis and Zone 1 lateral stenosis can be equally well demonstrated on water soluble myelograms and CT scans. Zone 2 stenosis is best demonstrated on CT scanning with neuroforamenal reconstructions. MR scanning is a promising alternative. CT reconstructions have a slight tendency to exaggerate the degree of stenosis secondary to bony changes in Zones 1 and 2 while not demonstrating the soft tissue component well. In contrast, the MR scan demonstrates the soft tissue changes well but minimizes the bony changes. If there has been previous surgery, the MR image can greatly exaggerate the degree of Zone 2 stenosis.

On occasion a patient who has peripheral neuropathy secondary to peripheral vascular disease, diabetes, or alcohol use will present with a mixed clinical picture suggestive of concomitant spinal stenosis. In this instance, EMG and nerve conduction tests can be of some help in sorting out which of the two conditions is the more significant clinically.

In the instance in which there appears to be almost exclusively a unilateral radicular process accounting for the patient's symptoms selective nerve root blocks have proven helpful in determining, with assurance, which nerve should receive the surgeons' primary attention.

All investigations must, however, be placed in the perspective of a careful history.

Treatment

Rest, flexion exercise, analgesics, nonsteroidal antiinflammatory drugs, and epidural steroid injections have a place in the medical management of the less severe of the spinal stenotic syndromes (Chap. 3). In our experience the results of epidural cortico-steroid injections are often excellent, albeit unpredictable. Well planned and carefully targeted surgical decompression remains the most important treatment modality in patients with significant disability. The question of "what constitutes significant disability" requires a careful discussion between patient and physician concerning the patient's needs and desires as contrasted with the risks and achievable goals of surgery.

Prognosis

As a byproduct of a recent study of stenosis patients who were treated with surgical decompression (Weinstein et al., 1983) it was noted that these patients experienced significant improvement at the two year follow-up. This should not give a false sense of value of this modality of treatment. Firstly, none of the patients were returned to a completely normal status by the surgery. The improvement from the preoperative status to the post operative status was about one half of the difference (on a numerical standard) between the preoperative value and normal. Secondly, with time this degree of improvement tends to deteriorate because of the inevitable progression of the degenerative process. For these reasons, and because the patients tend to be elderly, we try all of the above conservative modalities before suggesting surgery in most of our patients. The exceptions are the very severely affected and those with cauda equina syndrome. A reasonable rule of thumb for considering surgical treatment in patients with pseudoclaudication would be the inability to walk 200 meters without resting.

10 The patient with chronic low back pain

Introduction

Chronic low back pain is a term used, not to describe the severity of pain, but rather the time period during which a patient has had pain. Although the point in time at which pain becomes "chronic" is arbitrary, we use three months as our limit. This choice is because studies of the natural history of low back pain indicates that 90–95% recover within a three month period and also because patients with low back pain lasting for longer than three months have a poorer prognosis and pose the largest problems in terms of management and cost (Fig. 1). In epidemiologic studies chronic pain has been defined as (a) pain that persists beyond the normal healing time for an acute injury or disease, or (b) pain related to a chronic disease, or (c) pain that emerges and persists or recurs episodically for months or years (Bonica and Chapman, 1986).

As will be obvious when reading this chapter, acute and chronic pain are fundamentally different. While acute pain bears a direct relationship to peripheral stimulus, nociception and tissue damage, chronic pain becomes increasingly dissociated from its original physiological basis, with little or no objective evidence of nociceptive stimulus (Waddell, 1987). While pharmacological, physical and surgical treatment methods are highly successful in

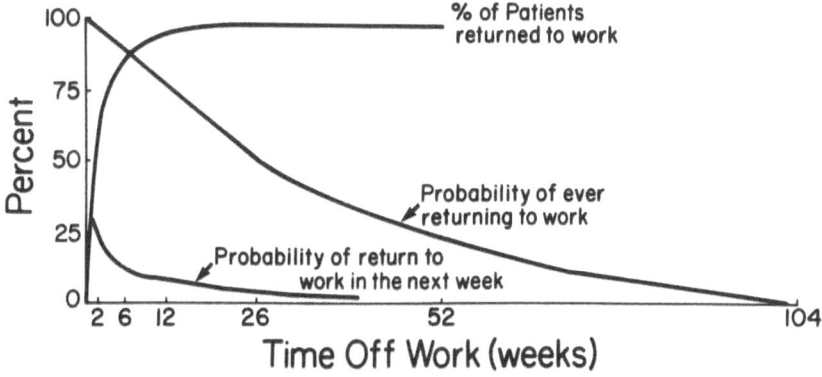

Fig. 1. Illustration of decrease in work return as a function of time

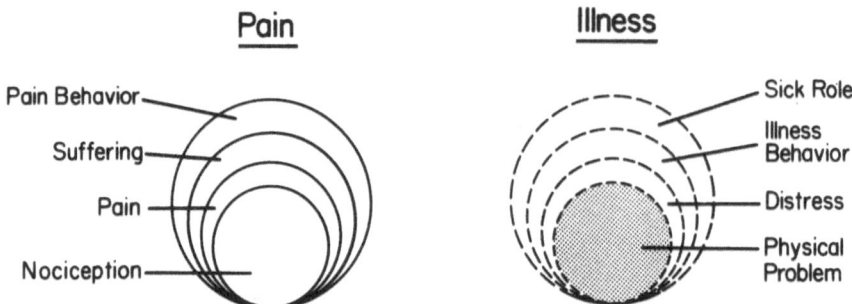

Fig. 2. Conceptual model of pain and illness. (Adapted from Waddell, 1987)

appropriate patients with acute pain, chronic pain is often resistant to such treatment. The patients no longer suffer from pain only but become emotionally distressed, depressed and develop a pain behaviour. The conceptual model of pain proposed by Loeser (1982) is useful to understand how pain changes from nociception to suffering and pain behaviour (Fig. 2). Chronic pain and disability should also be distinguished. They are not synonymous, but have a complex relationship. Pain is what the patient says he has, and is influenced by attitudes, beliefs, distress, and illness behaviour (Waddell et al., 1984). Disability is what patients say they can do thereby influenced by their interpretation of that word (usually as an injury), past experience, and advice on how to manage pain.

Waddell (1987) has suggested that a biopsychosocial concept of illness should be applied to clinical practice when managing patients with chronic low back pain. In his model, which is similar to Loeser's pain model, illness is emphasized rather than pain. The initial physical problems gradually become replaced by distress and illness behaviour and ultimately the patient adopts a sick role (Fig. 2).

The theories of chronic pain are important to the understanding of the patient with chronic back pain. They imply that there is no proportional relationship between the physical pathology and the patients presenting symptoms and disability. Clinical diagnosis, then, is not required for treatment and a fundamental pathological basis for rational physical treatment does not exist. A further discussion of this occurs in Chap. 13.

Differential diagnosis

Chronic low back pain, as defined above, is a symptom diagnosis, not a diagnosis based on etiology. Unfortunately chronic back patients do not present with a homogeneous symptom complex, but can be subdivided further into several groups using different subclassification systems. For example, chronic low back patients can be divided into those with organic findings, those with nonorganic findings and those with psychological findings. Chronic back patients have also been divided into those unable to work and those still working. From a syndrome point of view, they can also be divided into those with mechanically sensitive low back pain, those with continuous low back pain and those with inflammatory low back pain. A fourth syndrome group are patients with "chronic pain syndrome". These patients display symptoms of mechanically sensitive and/or continuous low back pain. They should be separated from those groups, however, because organic findings explaining their pain are rare and psychological and psychosocial factors have led to specific behaviour patterns. Classifying patients into these four groups is not always easy, and indeed sometimes patients move from group to group. In all groups, sciatica can occur as part of the patient's symptoms. The term chronic low back pain in this chapter includes those patients as well.

Mechanically sensitive back pain

Patients with mechanically sensitive back pain are separated from the other groups by the fact that their pain is so strongly dependent on whether or not they are loading their spines. The type of loading at which pain increases differs between patients. Some are particularly sensitive to loads occurring when lifting, bending and twisting. Others are more sensitive to prolonged static work postures, which limits the time period during which they can sit or stand. Others still have increased pain both in dynamic and static loading conditions. Most patients with chronic back pain fall into this last group, with some postural discomfort and increased pain with lifting, bending and twisting as well. These patients have often had an acute onset of their pain, not infrequently related to work. They have often been treated with passive treatment modalities, such as rest, heat or cold treatment, ultrasound and massage. They have either not been stimulated to return to work or are unable to do so because of the physical requirements of work and because light duty alternatives do not exist. Although physical findings do exist in these patients, they are often few, mainly restricted range of motion and positive straight leg raising which do not allow conclusions as to the etiology of the problem. A separate group with mechanically sensitive low back pain are patients with true sciatica secondary to herniated lumbar discs. These patients sometimes function remarkably well and are (almost) free of pain at rest. Many of these patients have made major lifestyle changes, avoiding activities that cause increased pain. As time goes on, however, they become increasingly frustrated (distressed) by these self imposed restrictions, seeking medical and surgical solutions to their problem. Careful examination will reveal the symptoms and signs discussed in Chap. 5.

Patients with spinal stenosis also fit into this group of patients. The characteristics of those patients have been discussed in Chap. 9. In these patients pain is often aggravated by standing, and claudication when walking is present in 50%.

Other diagnostic entities to look for in the chronic low back pain patients with mechanically sensitive symptoms include facet osteoarthritis and the facet syndrome (Mooney and Robertson, 1976), disc resorbtion and disc disruption (Crock, 1986), and segmental instability (Frymoyer and Selby, 1985). The facet syndrome is suggested in patients who have increased pain on hyperextension and when twisting. Radiographs and particularly CT-scans will demonstrate degenerative changes in the facet joints.

Disc disruption and segmental instability are both controversial diagnoses. In the case of disc disruption, which is probably quite rare, plane radiographs are often normal, and the patients pain quite persistent. In segmental instability degenerative changes are present along with traction spurs (osteophytes) and changes in the relationship between vertebraes on flexion-extension films. Using strict diagnostic criteria instability is probably quite uncommon.

Continuous low back pain

Patients with continuous low back pain and/or sciatica are quite rare. It is in this group that we find the patients with severe low back pain discussed in Chap. 9. It is also in this group that we find the malingering patient discussed in Chap. 13. Although patients with chronic pain syndrome more often belong to the group with mechanically sensitive back pain, they are also found in the group with continuous low back pain. The patients in this group, when asked about their pain, will say that it is continuous and unrelenting. It disturbs sleep and requires constant medication. Symptom amplification from mechanical loading can occur but from a base level of pain which is much higher than in the mechanically sensitive group. Organic findings are not uncommon among patients who have severe, unremitting low back pain of organic origin (Chap. 9). Nonorganic findings, on the other hand, are quite common among those who are malingering and psychological findings are quite common both among the malingerers and in the group with the chronic pain syndrome. It should be emphasized that true malingering is relatively uncommon. Therefore patients with chronic unrelenting pain should not be immediately classified as such (Chap. 13). Any back patient who presents with continuous severe pain should be considered as having an organic disease. Appropriate tests should be ordered or, if existing, reviewed. If no organic cause of the pain complaint is found, then the diagnosis of "chronic pain syndrome" or "malingering" can be considered.

Inflammatory back disease

Patients with inflammatory back disease frequently present with chronic pain lasting for several years. Men below age 40 are most commonly affected. Usually, pain is more severe in the early morning hours and accompanied by morning stiffness, while, both pain and stiffness improve over the day. Not infrequently, there will also be other expressions of the underlying disease since it is not confined to the spine only.

Chronic pain syndrome

The chronic pain syndrome is a term used to describe the situation in which an acute medical problem has transferred into one in which psychological and psychosocial factors gradually become the most important. It is important to differentiate the chronic pain syndrome from acute pain or recurring acute pain because the treatment of these three conditions is entirely different. The persistent treatment of chronic pain syndrome, as if it were an acute problem, is unsuccessful and leads to prolonged pain and sickness absence. In the worst of cases, treatment can in fact lead to complications which in themselves become exceedingly difficult to treat. An example of such is the multiply operated back with chronic arachnoiditis.

In the chronic pain syndrome, pain rarely serves a biological function. Therefore the classic medical treatment model becomes inappropriate. Physical findings are usually inconclusive and often non-organic in nature (Chap. 2). Psychological and environmental factors lead to the development of a "chronic pain behavior."

In a chronic pain syndrome patient pain gradually changes into suffering (Loeser and Black, 1975) (Fig. 2). It is important to the understanding of the chronic pain patient to recognize the difference between pain and suffering. Although suffering often occurs in the presence of pain, it is defined as a state of severe distress associated with events that threaten the intactness of the person (Cassell, 1982). Fordyce (1976) has termed the many observable manifestations of pain problems which are related to suffering as pain behaviours. These include abnormal physical positioning, excessive talk about pain, multiple physician visits, unemployment, excessive bed rest, limping, wincing, crying and inappropriate medication. All of these pain behaviours are further reinforced by psychosocial problems. These patients are usually quite frustrated, having undergone a number of physical examinations and diagnostic procedures without definitive diagnosis. They become preoccupied with their pain, which becomes the central focus of their lives. This can result in hostility, in loss of friends and in disruption of family relationships (Addison, 1984, 1985). Waddell (1987), in his biopsychosocial model talks about illness behaviour, instead of pain behaviour, defined as "observable and potentially measurable actions and conduct which expresses and communicates the individual's own perception of disturbed health" (Waddell et al., 1984) (Fig. 2). Illness, then, is considered a social phenomenon rather than a disease.

Diagnostics

In spite of the fact that patients with chronic low back pain often have been extensively investigated in the past, it is quite important to obtain a thorough patient history, and to perform a detailed clinical examination. This will not only make the patient aware of the fact that you are actively seeking a diagnosis, but will also allow you to differentiate between chronic pain of organic nature and chronic pain of a nonorganic nature. The work-up should be done as a single definite attempt. It is obviously useful to have access to previous work-up and conclusions. Access to previous diagnostic tests will save time and money and can be used for comparative purposes if new tests are indicated.

The patient history should follow the general concept outlined in Chap. 2. Information about precipitating events, work relatedness, previous injuries and the patient's description of the original pain and of changes in pain are all important. It should be attempted to find out which effect pain has on the patient emotionally and how the patient sees his or her future with respect to treatment and work.

The physical examination serves to exclude organic findings conclusive to a specific diagnosis. Patients with severe unremitting low back pain must be studied with particular care. The non-organic physical signs should be tested for in all patients with chronic back pain (Table 1). Pain drawings are very helpful since the way patients draw their pain and other symptoms is influenced by distress.

The main problem in the diagnostic work-up of patients with low back pain is to decide the extent to which structural and other diagnostic procedures should be pursued. In our opinion, standard radiographs should always be obtained in a patient with chronic low back pain if they are not already available. Repeating standard X-rays is not indicated. If spinal instability is suspected, flexion-extension films can be helpful. In patients where a disc herniation (Chap. 5) or spinal stenosis (Chap. 9) are suspected, computerized axial tomographs should be obtained at this point if not already available. With negative radiographs and a negative CT, we do not feel that there is any indication for a magnetic resonance study unless signs and symptoms indicative of infectious disease or tumor exists. A myelogram should only be obtained when surgery is being contemplated. Radionucleide

Table 1. A comparison of the symptoms and signs of physical disease and abnormal illness behaviour in chronic low-back pain

	Physical disease/ normal illness behaviour	Magnified or inappropriate illness behaviour
Pain drawing	localized neuroanatomic proportionate	nonanatomic regional magnified
Pain adjectives	sensory	emotional
Symptoms		
pain	localized	whole leg pain tailbone pain
numbness	dermatomal	whole leg numbness
weakness	myotomal	whole leg giving way
time pattern	varies with time	never free of pain
response to treatment	variable benefit	intolerance of treatments emergency admission to hospital
Signs		
tenderness	localized	superficial, widespread, nonanatomic
axial loading	no lumbar pain	lumbar pain
simulated rotation	no lumbar pain	lumbar pain
straight leg raising	limited on distraction	improves with distraction
sensory	dermatomal	regional
motor	myotomal	regional, jerky, giving way
general response	appropriate pain	overreaction

scanning is only indicated if bone disease, inflammatory changes or a tumor are diagnostic possibilities. Neurodiagnostics are only indicated when radiculopathy exists, and laboratory procedures can be reduced to obtaining an ESR for purposes of excluding infection, inflammation and tumor. Thus, in the majority of patients history, physical examination and standard radiographs are sufficient.

Psychological tests are helpful in patients with chronic back pain. A more extensive discussion of these tests is presented in Chap. 13.

Treatment

Treatment should be specific when an organic cause of chronic low back pain is present. It has been established that even in patients who have significant psychological disturbances, and chronic pain behaviour, treatment of the

Table 2. Treatment objectives in chronic low back pain syndrome

Objectives
1. One comprehensive evaluation
2. Active physical treatment
3. Avoid excess treatment
4. Avoid creating dependence
5. Exercise
6. Education and behaviour modification

underlying organic cause of the disease will reverse this problem and result in an excellent outcome. In patients with chronic back pain without specific organic cause, it is important to remember than many treatment modalities which are applicable to acute low back pain are contraindicated (Table 2). Medication should be reduced to minimal levels. This often requires a detoxification procedure since the patients are psychologically addicted. Only acetaminophen, or aspirin and/or nonsteroidal antiinflammatory drugs should be prescribed. Medication taken "as needed", should be discouraged, and replaced by a specific dosage program. Antidepressants are useful in some of these patients as discussed in Chap. 3.

Bedrest is discouraged. Short rest periods, decreasing rapidly to no rest periods at all are recommended. While there is some support for a short period of bedrest in acute pain, as discussed in Chap. 3, there is absolutely no support in chronic back pain. On the contrary, bedrest has several negative effects, including a decrease in physical fitness, a demineralization of bone, a loss in muscle strength and mass, a general feeling of malaise, increased physical distress and depression, loss of work habit, loss of job opportunity and a decreased probability of returning to work (Waddell, 1987). The use of corsets and braces should also be discouraged and instead physical therapy should be started. This therapy must be active, relying on patient participation. Contrary to what many patients perceive, exercise does not have to increase pain. Its positive physiological effects are undisputed, including effects on bone, muscle, cartilage, tendon and disc. Exercise also increases endorphine levels, reduces sensitivity to pain, and promotes return to work. Exercise methods that terminate "at tolerance levels" should not be used, since they tend to increase pain behaviour. This is because of the strong influence of conscious feedback on how much exercise has been done. Rather, the so-called "working to quota" method is more successful in these patients, probably because of decreased anxiety. Working to quota is defined as working to a level of activity that is less than the level at which pain occurs. After a period of working to a certain quota, the activity level (quota) is increased gradually. If pain occurs, then the quota is also reduced. Verbal praise and reinforcement markedly improves the exercise tolerance.

Education is also important in the treatment of chronic low back pain. Rehabilitation is made easier by the patient's appreciation of many of the facts discussed in this chapter relating to pain, suffering, distress and disability. Administered individually or as back-schools, patient education reduces fear and improves the patients' ability to deal with their situation. They can then take a more active role in their own rehabilitation.

Psychological treatment methods are quite important in the treatment of chronic low back pain syndrome. Behaviour modification by reinforcement of wellness behaviour with operant conditioning and with relaxation techniques, desensitization and assertiveness training have all been successfully used in the treatment of the patient with chronic pain syndrome. Behavioral treatment is not a single modality, but rather a concept by which pain is analyzed in terms of behaviour and then it is attempted to change that behaviour. It involves reducing medication and health care utilization, increased activity and modifying the family response to pain behaviour (Fordyce, 1976). The most powerful way to help a person change behaviour is by contingent reinforcement.

Work hardening has proved to be as particularly effective in returning patients to the working environment (Mayer et al., 1986). By active exercises combined with psychologic support and education, all patients in Mayer's et al. study increased their functional capacity (objectively measured), had less pain, less distress and 86% returned to work.

Summary

The key to chronic back pain is prevention. By actively treating acute pain, the development of the chronic pain syndrome can be avoided. In our opinion, most patients with chronic low back pain suffer because they have not been aggressively treated in the early stages of disease. By continuing to treat a chronic back patient as if he has acute disease, pain and disability are actually prolonged. The treatment of patients with chronic pain syndrome often requires a combination of several different treatment modalities.

11 The adult patient with spine deformity and low back pain

Introduction

The adult spine has a normal series of curves in the median (midsagittal) plane. The convex anterior cervical and lumbar curves are referred to as "lordosis" while the thoracic curve which is concave anteriorly is called "kyphosis". The normal ranges for these curves have significant variability. The normal thoracic kyphosis (as measured from the end plate of T-1 to T-12) is about 35° ($+/-$ 10°) and the normal lumbar lordosis (as measured from S-1 to L-1) is about 50° ($+/-$ 10°). The normal spine is straight in the frontal (coronal) plane.

Spinal deformity is a term used when a normal spine curvature is abnormally large or small, and when abnormal curvatures exist. It is also used to describe other types of abnormal structural relationships in the spine, such

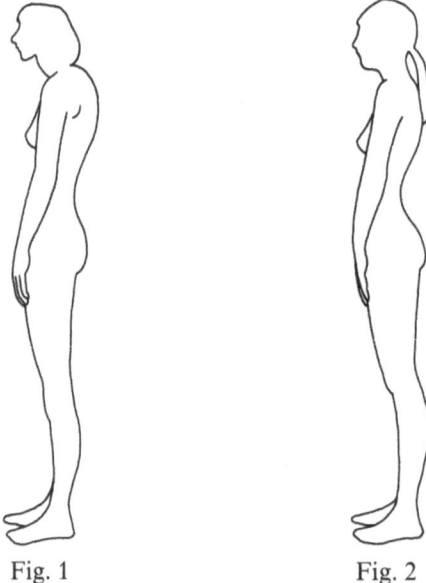

Fig. 1   Fig. 2

Fig. 1. A patient with excessive kyphosis

Fig. 2. A patient with excessive lordosis

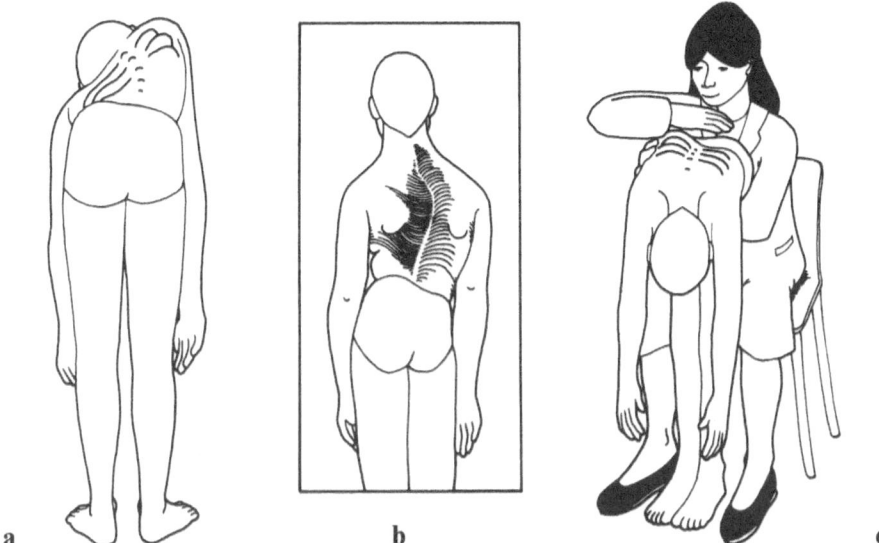

Fig. 3. Scoliosis. A severe posterior humping of ribs (**a**), which is secondary to vertebral body rotation (**b**). **c** When examining a patient with scoliosis a difference in height of the two sides of the posterior thorax can easily be seen when the patient bends over

as translational or rotational. Further it is used to describe abnormalities in spine development as described below. Spinal deformity is not a single entity and deformity per se and it is not a cause of lower back pain in most instances. Spine deformity is most easily classified on the basis of the plane of the deformity: (1) a deformity in the sagittal plane resulting in an abnormal increase in flexion is a *kyphotic* deformity (Fig. 1); (2) a deformity in the median plane resulting in an abnormal increase in extension is a *lordotic* deformity (Fig. 2); (3) a deformity in the frontal plane with an abnormal side bending of the spine is a *scoliosis* or a *scoliotic* deformity (Fig. 3); (4) a deformity in which one vertebra is displaced in relation to the adjacent vertebra, is a *translational* deformity; (5) a deformity about the axis of the spine is a *rotational* deformity or a *shortening* deformity; (6) deformities of the structure of individual vertebra occur both in the shape of the vertebra itself as is seen in *congenital scoliosis* (Chap. 12) with wedging and in the internal dimensions of the neural canal as in *spinal stenosis* (see Chap. 9).

History

In the analysis of problems of spinal deformity as a cause of lower back pain one must determine the age of onset or first discovery of the deformity and the temporal relationship of the deformity to the onset of pain. The date of discovery may not be the actual date of origin, since patients and their families are often unaware of minor deformities, and not infrequently even of major ones. One must be careful to determine the character of the pain, e.g. is it mechanical or radicular, persistent or intermittent, present or absent at night, etc. (Chap. 2). These facts are important since they will help to elucidate the etiology of the deformity and suggest whether the pain is originating from the structural elements or the neural elements.

So called "mechanical" back pain is of three types: (1) The sudden onset of severe lower back pain which is constant, aggravated by any motion, and associated with prominent spasm is typical of the sudden failure of a structural element (see Chap. 4); (2) Recurrent attacks of lower back pain (see Chap. 5); and (3) Low back pain associated with stiffness, gelling and aggravation by moderate to heavy activity (see Chap. 10).

Symptoms arising from injury or irritation of the neural elements will give rise to complaints of numbness, parasthesias, weakness, pain, and occasionally can cause sphincter disturbance. These complaints may be absent in patients with back pain and spinal deformity or they may constitute the entire syndrome as in patients who are unaware of a translational deformity when they present with a lumbar radiculopathy.

Physical examination

The physical examination requires careful attention to the patients posture as viewed from the front, back, side and with the patient flexed at the waist (Chap. 2). From the anterior view the spinal deformity can be represented by shortened trunk height as compared with limb length, a protuberant abdo-

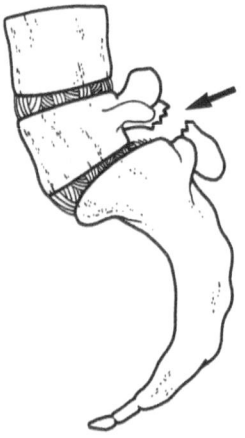

Fig. 4. Spondylolisthesis

men in the absence of obesity, and chest deformity. Deformity of the chest with decreased height and increased A-P diameter is characteristic of kyphosis (Winter et al., 1973), while a protuberant abdomen suggests an increased lordosis. Asymmetric chest deformity suggests scoliosis. The deformity associated with a significant degree of lower lumbar spondylolisthesis is best appreciated in the lateral view, with the appearance of normal chest proportions and shortening of the interval between the chest and pelvis (Wiltse, 1962). Often there is a "step off" at the lumbosacral junction (Fig. 4). The lateral view also gives the best perspective of kyphosis and lordosis. The view from posterior and both with the patient upright and flexed at the waist are best for the detection of a scoliotic deformity. Lateral trunk shift as measured with a plumb line and rib or paraspinal muscular elevations are indicative of rotation of the spine, which occurs in conjunction with scoliosis (except the relatively unusual congenital variety). Most scoliotic deformities are complex combinations of lateral bending, rotation, and alterations in lordosis and kyphosis which are beyond the scope of this discussion.

Pathology

Spinal deformities can also be classified on the basis of the etiology of the deformity. *Congenital* deformity of the spine may be due to hereditary factors or intrauterine injury. These include many combinations of partial or complete failure of segmentation and/or deletions of spinal components. *Infectious* diseases are a notorious cause of deformity (see Chap. 15). Both benign and malignant *tumorous* conditions can result in spinal deformity (see Chap. 15). *Inflammatory* diseases of some types produce progressive kyphosis and often begin as chronic lower back pain (see Chap. 16). *Developmental* spinal deformities such as adolescent kyphosis or "idiopathic" scoliosis are common spinal deformities in which the true etiology is only partially understood. *Degenerative* diseases can result in spinal deformity in later life (Chap. 9) while *neurologic* diseases may result in early severe deformity if present while the patient is growing and to a lesser extent after growth is completed. *Metabolic* diseases may produce significant spinal deformity with significant secondary pain problems. The most important metabolic disease in this context is osteoporosis (see Chap. 17). *Trauma* produces spinal deformity when there is disruption of structural elements. Fractures, for example, can produce deformity by asymmetrical crushing of bone or by tearing of ligaments with secondary deformity under conditions of loading by gravity or muscular activity. *Psychological* disturbance such as conversion hysteria can present as both pain and deformity (see Chap. 13).

The problem, as presented, at first seems complex; however, the presumed mechanisms of pain production in each of these types of deformity are the same. First, the cause of the deformity may be a destructive process such as tumor, infection, inflammatory disease, or trauma each of which is a potential cause of pain in and of itself. Secondly, the deformity may result in abnormal loads being carried by the structural elements of the spine leading to failure of one or several of these elements, which may become painful. Thirdly, the deformity may lead to injury of visceral structures resulting in potentially painful conditions.

Adult scoliosis and spondylolisthesis

Spondylolisthesis and adult scoliosis are two specific types of spinal deformity of special interest. In the majority of patients with adult scoliosis or spondylolisthesis the condition is not painful. In fact, the incidence of low back pain in adults with scoliosis is the same as in the unaffected (by scoliosis) population (Weinstein, 1986; Nachemson, 1968). However, when pain occurs it is more severe, more persistent and more likely to result in disability (Jackson et al., 1983). Lumbar curves are more likely to be painful than higher curves. A similar situation holds in spondylolisthesis (Bosworth et al., 1955; Laurent, 1978). Spondylolisthesis can result in pain at any time after its onset, which is usually between the ages of six and eighteen (Chap. 12). However, the more usual situation is for the less common severe degrees of slip to present in adolescence while the lesser degrees (under 33%) of slip may never become symptomatic; or, should symptoms occur they develop in middle adult life (Wiltse, 1977).

Patients with adult scoliosis usually do not have pain; however, when pain does occur there are three identifiable syndromes (Kostuick, 1979; Simmons and Jackson, 1979; Jackson et al., 1983). In the younger adult, the pain associated with a lumbar scoliosis usually occurs at about the apex of the curve. This is thought to be related to either disc degeneration at this level or to chronic muscular fatigue. In the older adult, the symptoms are more likely to be lower in the curve or in the lumbar compensatory curve. This is thought to be a result of the abnormal stresses on the facet joints and discs resulting in an accelerated and more severe degenerative process. The third syndrome is radicular in nature and is the result of nerve root entrapment on the concave side of the curve in zone 2 of the neuroforamen (Simmons and Jackson, 1979) (see Chap. 9). This comes about either from gradual progression of the curve in adult life or from asymmetrical disc degeneration and collapse resulting in subluxation of the superior facet into the neuroforamen (VanDam et al., 1987; Swank et al., 1981).

The presumed mechanism of pain in the adult with spondylolisthesis is quite similar to that in the adult with scoliosis (Lusskin, 1965; Wiltse, 1977). The onset of symptoms of lower back pain correlates well with the onset of disc degeneration and, thus, is considered "discogenic" in nature. The second syndrome is that of radicular pain which is most often (in the moderate degrees of slipping) due to entrapment of the root passing under the spondylolytic defect at the level of the pars interarticularis. The space under the pars is decreased by the accumulation of fibrous tissue around the defect, collapse of the neuroforamen due to discal narrowing, and an "elephant foot" excressence of bone at the level of the pseudarthrosis of the pedicle.

Spondylolisthesis may occur in adults secondary to severe degeneration of the three joint complex in the lumbar spine. This most often occurs at the L4-L5 level and is more common in women. This "degenerative spondylolisthesis" causes a secondary spinal stenosis which is central and may produce symptoms of pseudo claudication (see Chap. 9) or an individual nerve root entrapment (Rosenberg, 1976).

Kyphosis

An adolescent in whom there has been the gradual onset of increasing thoracic kyphosis which was mildly painful from the beginning (Scheuermann's kyphosis; see Chap. 12) can develop lower back pain as a secondary event (Ogilvie and Sherman, 1987). Two different causes of pain are presumed to be present in this example. The Scheuermann's deformity is thought to be a form of adolescent osteoporosis (Bradford et al., 1975, 1976, 1980; Lusskin, 1965) in which there is progressive wedging of the bone and protrusion of disc material into the softened bone. These dynamic changes produce the back ache in the area of deformity which is most often thoracic. As a secondary effect of the increased thoracic kyphosis (greater than 45°) there is an increase in lumbar lordosis (greater than 60°). Third in the chain of events is an increased load on the L-5 pars interarticularis. This increased load, if large enough, can result in a stress fracture of the pars which may become chronic (spondylolysis). This may result in lower back pain (Chap. 12).

An elderly woman may have noticed the progressive kyphosis due to osteoporosis with loss of height and intermittent severe pain in either the thoracic or lumbar spine (see Chap. 17). In this instance the progressive depletion of the amount of vertebral bone results in such weakening that at some point the bone is unable to carry the normal loads of gravity and activity. This may result in a mildly painful gradual deformity (dowager's hump) or in a sudden collapse with severe pain (compression fracture).

Investigations

The investigations which are necessary in patients presenting with symptomatic spinal deformity must first be directed toward the diagnosis of the etiology of the deformity such as metabolic, developmental, etc.; and second-ly, to potential site of radicular symptoms when present. In any instances the initial studies must include standard radiographs. The need for additional studies will be determined by the etiology which has been suggested by the radiographs, the presence or absence of radicular symptoms, the severity of the symptoms, and the response to the initial therapy (see Chaps. 2 and 6).

Treatment

The appropriate choice for treatment in spinal deformity with associated lower back pain and/or radicular symptoms is dependent upon the etiology of the deformity and the location and severity of associated nerve injury or irritation. Spinal deformity is a condition for the specialist and patients with such should be referred for evaluation and further treatment. Most deformi-ties can, to some degree, be prevented when detected early and treated appropriately. This will prevent development of severe complex syndromes with sometimes life-threatening complications.

12 Back pain in children

Contributed by R. N. Hensinger

Introduction

Low back pain is not a common complaint of childhood, and when children do complain of such pain the probability of serious pathology is far greater than when adults have similar complaints. Therefore, each instance of low back pain in a pediatric practice must be evaluated with great care.

In 1980, at the University of Michigan, a survey of one-hundred childred with back pain revealed that all but 15 % had a definite identifiable cause for their complaint. A remarkable 18 % had either tumor or infection, and approximately 33% were found to have a post traumatic cause such as an occult fracture or spondylolysis/spondylolisthesis. An additional third of the children were found to have developmental problems, usually kyphosis or scoliosis. It is important to note that the cause for the complaint was often not evident on the first visit, and that often extensive diagnostic work was required.

History

The history obtained from the parents of very young children may be very non-specific and may be nothing more than a recent refusal to walk or the development of a postural change. Even older children provide considerable difficulty for the examiner as they are often not able to localize their musculoskeletal complaints. They tend to be expansive with their gestures often indicating the entire back rather than an area such as the lumbosacral junction. Thus, it is necessary to spend the extra time to elicit the important historical points.

Trauma is commonly described by children and their parents or guardian. A traumatic origin of pain, however, should not immediately be accepted at face value. Care must be taken to discover the true extent of the trauma or injury, its mechanism and severity, and the temporal relationship to the onset of symptoms. If the onset of the pain is during athletics such as gymnastics, weight lifting, or the butterfly stroke in swimming, then either spondylolysis/spondylolisthesis or apophyseal injury should be excluded (Jackson et al., 1976; Handel et al., 1979; Keller, 1974; Lippitt, 1976; Lowrey, 1973; Micheli,

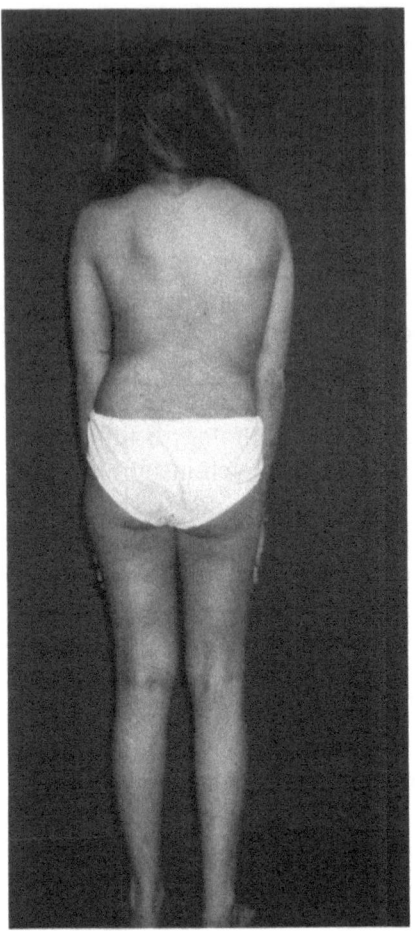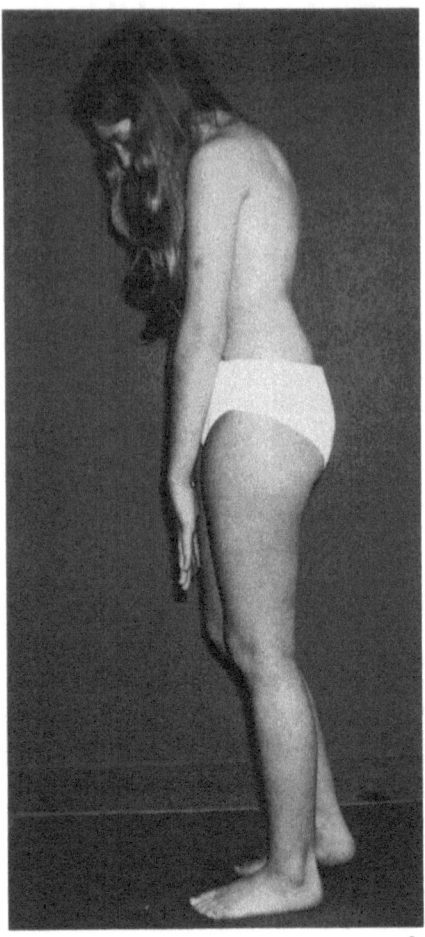

a   b

Fig. 1. Twelve year old with spondylolysis/spondylolisthesis demonstrating clinically
a scoliosis, and **b** the tightness of the hamstrings markedly restricts forward bending.
c Anterior-posterior and **d** lateral roentgenograms demonstrate a 35° scoliosis and
Grade II spondylolisthesis. Symptoms and physical findings resolved completely with
surgical stabilization of L5-S1

1979; Techakapuch, 1981). A family history of spondylolisthesis (Hensinger
et al., 1976) is also helpful as there is a high rate of occurrence of this
condition among family members and among certain ethnic groups.

Specific note should be taken of relief by aspirin and night pain as these
are suggestive of osteoid osteoma or osteoblastoma (Keim and Reima, 1975;
Kirwan et al., 1984; Mehta and Murray, 1977). Morning stiffness associated
with lower back pain is suggestive of ankylosing spondylitis. Here again
aspirin may provide some degree of consistent relief.

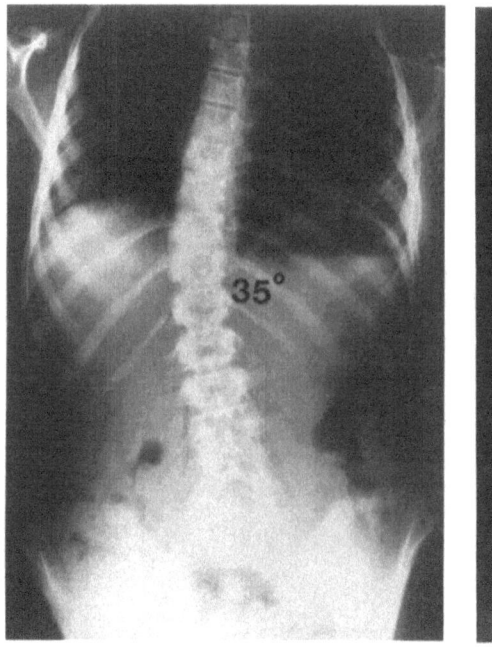
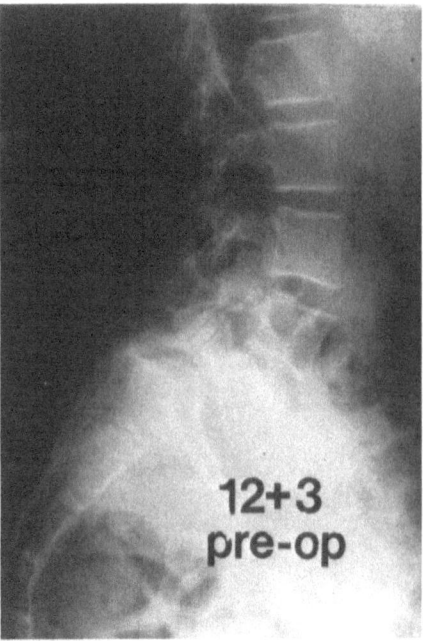

c   d

The dangerous signs of childhood back pain are persistent pain unrelieved by rest or immobilization, increasing pain, unexplainted fever, and
symptoms of systemic illness such as malaise and weight loss. Patients with
spinal neoplasm or infection may also present with abdominal pain and
guarding.

Complaints referable to the nervous system are uncommon in children
and demand special attention. Radicular pain, parasthesias, weakness, foot
deformity, and change in sphincter control in a previously continent child
(including the last onset of enuresis) suggest that a very serious problem may
be in progress demanding immediate evaluation (Fig. 2a).

Scoliosis

The history of pain associated with scoliosis and/or a left thoracic curve
suggests neoplasm, adolescent kyphosis (Scheuermann's disease), infection,
or spondylolisthesis. One should never accept "scoliosis" as the cause of
back pain in a child until all serious causes have been eliminated. It is a
practical 'rule of thumb' that scoliosis per se is not a cause of pain in children
(Figs. 1 and 2).

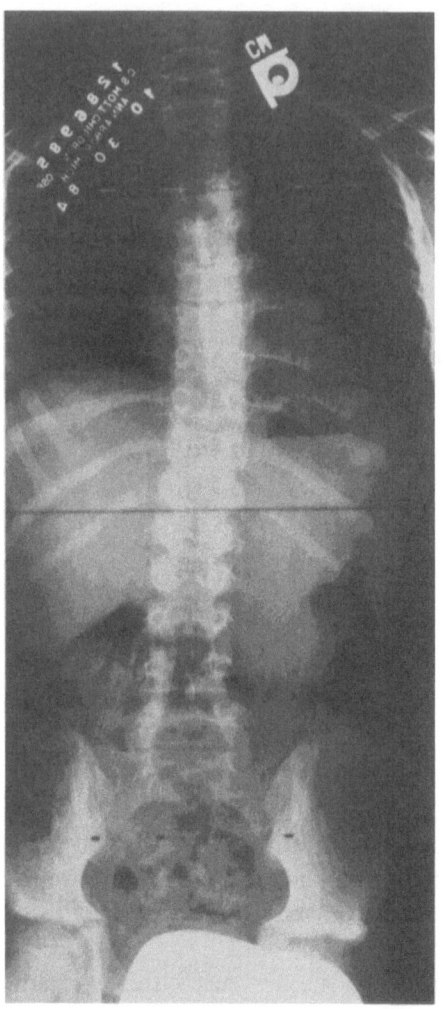

a

Fig. 2. Seven year old with back pain due to an osteoblastoma. **a** The routine roentgenograms demonstrate a mild scoliosis, but the lesion could not be identified on this view. **b** The bone scan demonstrates increased uptake of the isotope in the region of L4–5 on the right. **c** CT scan demonstrates lesion in pedicle L5

Physical examination

It is important that the focus of the examination is not narrowed too early and remains broad during the evaluation. The immature spine is quite flexible and simple guarding or posturing due to a painful lesion can result in an alarming degree of scoliosis (Fig. 1a). Hamstring tightness may be so severe that the child is unable to bend at the waist (Fig. 1b).

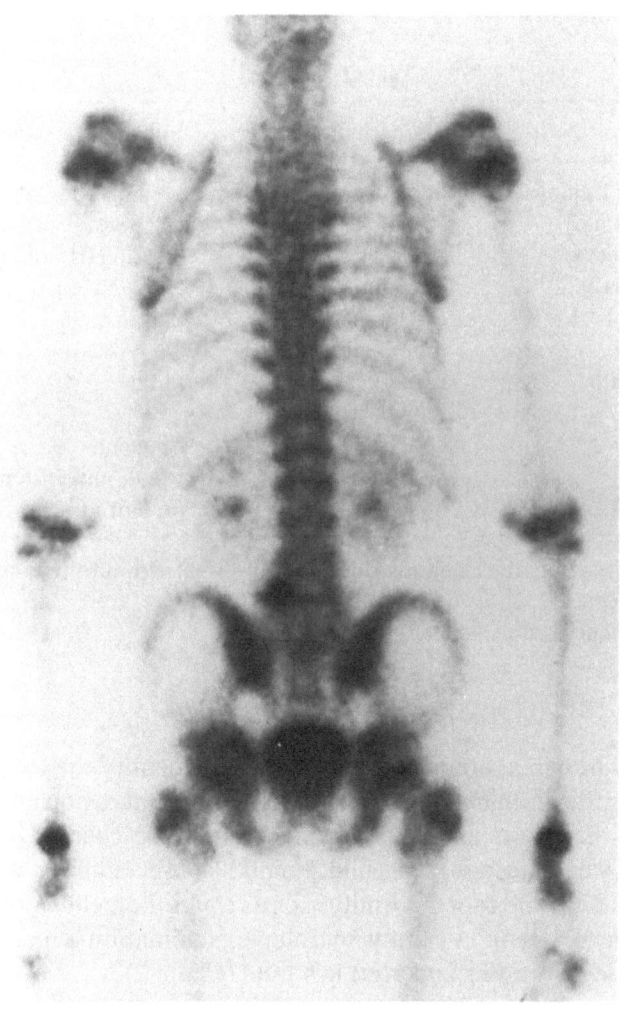

b

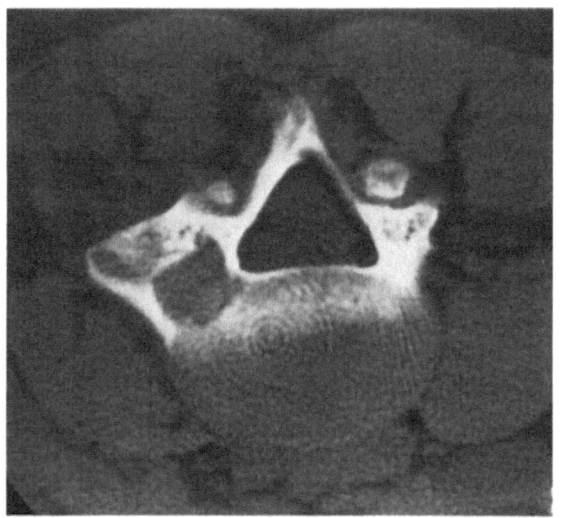

c

Table 1. Scoliosis

	Idiopathic	Infection or neoplasm
1. Neurologic findings	none	possible
2. Family history	80%	negative
3. Age of onset*	**8 +	ALL CHILDREN
4. Curve patterns	right thoracic	*may have left
	left lumbar	thoracic
	thoracolumbar	
5. Progression	variable	rapid
	growth dependent	
6. Pain	none	frequent
7. Sex	80–90% female	equal, male = female
8. Cafe au lait	none	present in neurofibromatosis

* Rare infantile idiopathic scoliosis does exist in Great Britain predominantly and may be left thoracic
** Congenital curves do exist

Palpation or percussion of the spine can help identify the localization of the lesion in spite of an unspecific history. The inguinal region and the space between the iliac crest and lumbar spine should be checked for fullness suggestive of a cold abscess. The child should be observed when walking and for weakness, limp and foot deformity such as cavus foot, club foot, equinuus gait or atrophy of a limb. A careful neurologic examination is mandatory and should include Babinski's and Kernig's tests (Chap. 2).

Congenital anomalies

Congenital anomalies may be associated with back pain, such as diastematomyelia, dermoid cysts, lipomas of the cord, and tight filum terminale. Cutaneous abnormalities – hairy patches, nevi and dermal sinuses – are often (74%) associated with an underlying intraspinal anomaly (Gillespie et al., 1973; Hood et al., 1980; McMaster, 1984; Winter and Lipscomb, 1978). Similarly, a neurologic deficit is a common accompaniment (65%) but in children this may be a subtle finding, such as limping, thinness and/or shortness of the lower extremity, unilateral clubfoot, recurrent clubfoot, and urinary incontinence (McMaster, 1984). Spina bifida occulta with widening of the interpedicular distance and narrowing of the disc spaces is nearly always present at the site of an intraspinal anomaly. In diastematomyelia, a bony spur may be identified on the plain films, but will need myelographic confirmation.

Kyphosis: lumbar and dorsolumbar Scheuermann's disease

Scheuermann's disease is a common cause of thoracic kyphosis in the adolescent. The condition usually is not but can occasionally be mildly painful. The children commonly present with a deformity, and are subsequently found to have vertebral changes. Sorensen's (1964) radiographic criteria have been generally accepted to confirm the diagnosis, and include three or more adjacent vertebrae wedged more than 5°. Endplate irregularity, Schmorl's node formation, and narrowing of the disc space are common accompaniments, but are not in themselves diagnostic (Bradford et al., 1974).

Similar changes in the lumbar or dorsolumbar spine are less common, but more often accompanied by back pain (Greene et al., 1985). The condition can be encountered at any site, however it is most often localized to the dorsolumbar junction (Fig. 4), and usually affects more than one level (Hilton et al., 1976; Micheli, 1979). Several authors, including Scheuermann, suggest that the lumbar changes are more often the result of trauma, in contrast to the typical thoracic Scheuermann's disease which is spontaneous and more likely hereditary. Clinically it is accompanied by a period (2–6 months) of moderately severe pain with activity and a history of acute strain or injury (Greene et al., 1985). The symptoms are usually accentuated by forward flexion, and relieved by rest (Greene et al., 1985). Lumbar Scheuermann's is found twice as often in boys than in girls (Greene et al., 1985). Many investigators have noted a relationship between lumbar Scheuermann's disease and hard physical labor in immature teenagers (Greene et al., 1985; Scheuermann, 1961; Wiltse et al., 1975). More recently, Micheli (1979) found the condition to be more common than expected in young athletes, suggesting that the problem represents an injury to the vertebral growth plates.

The apophyseal ring is thinner in its center than at the periphery, and with increased pressure the intervertebral disc can be forced through the endplate and into cancellous bone with narrowing of the disc space (Resnick and Niwayama, 1978). Endplate rupture has been produced in the laboratory by compressing intervertebral motion segments, and is believed to be analogous to the mechanism that leads to Schmorl's nodes (Jayson et al., 1973). Heavy lifting, and bending increase dramatically the interdiscal pressure (Chap. 1). Micheli (1979) noted that the load on the spine occurring during the flexion-extension increments seen with rowers, weightlifters, and gymnasts (Fig. 5a, b) approaches the lower end of the range demonstrated experimentally to induce vertebral endplate fractures (Jayson et al., 1973). The findings of Greene et al. (1985) further support a traumatic etiology.

In some children the disc material passes peripherally (usually anterior), submarginally beneath the apophyseal ring (Greene et al., 1985) (Fig. 6a). Radiologically there will be separation of a triangular, smooth bone fragment

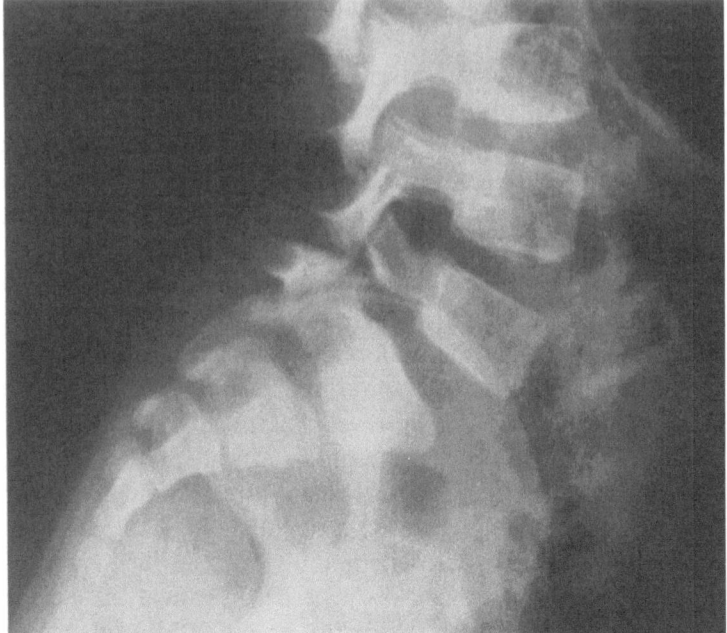

a

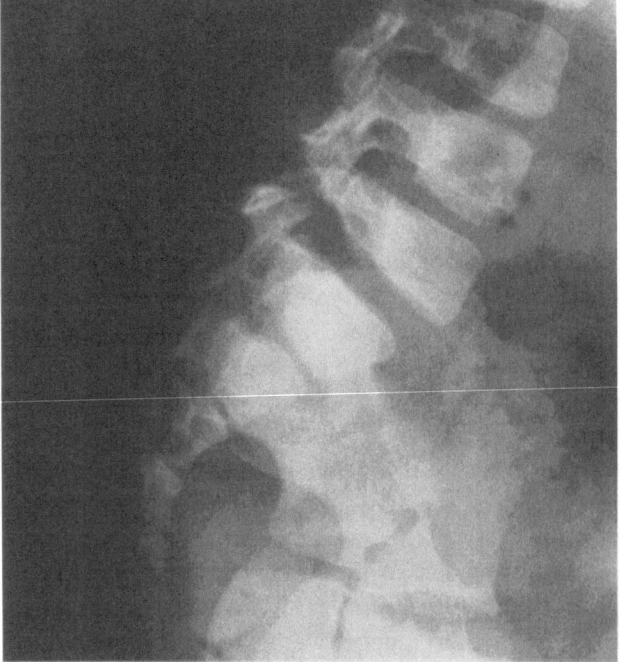

b

Fig. 3 a, b. Flexion-extension views of the lumbosacral junction in a nine year old demonstrating a spondylolysis and instability of this joint

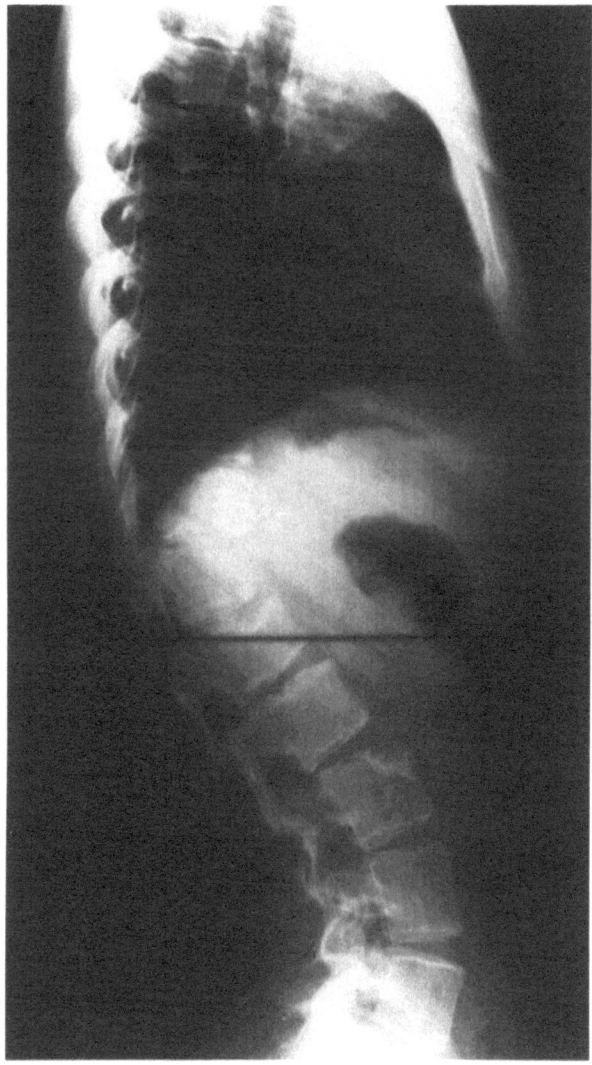

Fig. 4. Fourteen year old demonstrating severe kyphosis at the dorsolumbar junction, secondary to lumbar Scheuermann's disease. Note the endplate changes, wedging, and narrowing of the disc spaces. Schmorl's node formation can be seen as well in adjacent lumbar vertebrae

from the vertebral body which represents the ring apophysis. Radiographically this has been called "limbus vertebra". The vertebral changes progress slowly toward healing during the time of remaining growth (Fig. 6b). However, the Schmorl's node formation and disc space narrowing generally persists and the fragment of the ring apophysis typically remains separate from the vertebral body (Fig. 6b).

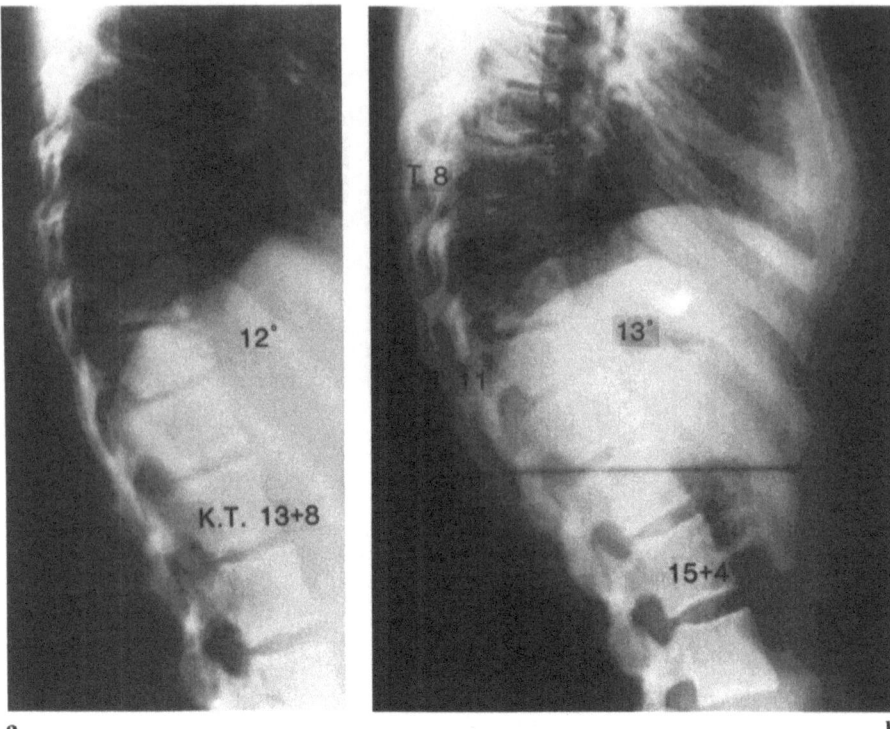

a   b

Fig. 5. Thirteen year old with **a** wedging and endplate changes at T11 secondary to gymnastics. **b** Note partial healing at one year, but no significant change in the degree of wedging. (Reproduced with permission from Rockwood CA, Wilkins KE, King RE (eds) Fractures in children. J. B. Lippincott, Philadelphia, 1984)

The majority of symptomatic teenagers respond quickly to simple rest and immobilization in a canvas corset or plastic orthosis (Greene et al., 1985; Micheli, 1979). Rarely will the deformity or symptoms be so severe as to require operative correction and stabilization.

Spondylolysis/spondylolisthesis

Spondylolysis in children occurs after walking age but rarely before five years of age and more commonly at seven or eight years (Baker and McHollick, 1956; Wiltse et al., 1975), which suggests that trauma is an important factor in the etiology. Although the history of minor trauma is common, and often initiates the onset of symptoms, the injury would seldom be classified as severe (Dandy and Shannon, 1971; Hensinger et al., 1976; Turner and Bianco, 1971). Rather, the onset of symptoms are insidious and coincide closely

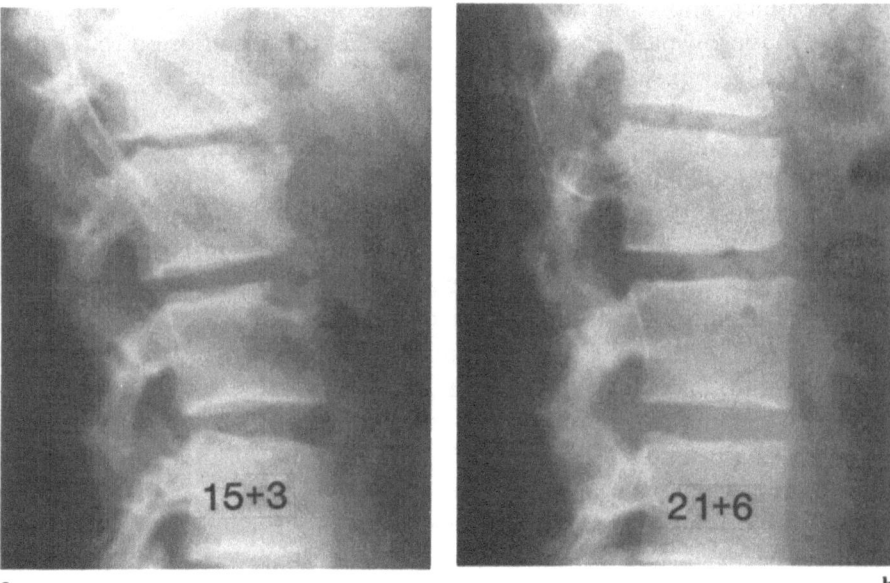

a   b

Fig. 6. a Fifteen year old with Schmorl's node formation and disc space narrowing secondary to weightlifting. Symptoms resolved completely with conservative treatment. Note the separation of a triangular bone fragment from the vertebral body, which represents the ring apophysis. **b** Roentgenogram at age 21 years demonstrating partial healing

with the adolescent growth spurt (Dandy and Shannon, 1971; Turner and Bianco, 1971).

Wiltse et al. (1975) suggest that spondylolysis represents a "stress" or fatigue fracture of the pars interarticularis. It is postulated that lumbar lordosis is accentuated by the normal hip flexion contractures of childhood. This posture focuses the forces of weightbearing on the pars interarticularis, leading to fatigue failure (Krentz and Troup, 1973). Laboratory studies suggest that shear stresses are greater on the pars interarticularis when the spine is extended, and further accentuated by lateral flexion movements on the extended spine, as may occur during a back walkover in gymnastics (Jackson et al., 1976). Jackson and coworkers noted that the incidence of spondylolysis was four times higher (11%) than expected in female gymnasts, some of whom initially had normal roentgenograms. Acute spondylolysis has been documented in soldiers who carry heavy backpacks and who perform exercises to which they are unaccustomed (Wiltse et al., 1975). Green and coworkers (1985) have noted a 35 percent incidence of spondylolysis in children with lumbar Scheuermann's disease, which is frequently accompanied by increased lumbar lordosis.

The pain in children with spondylolysis and spondylolisthesis is generally localized to the low back and, to a lesser extent, to the posterior buttocks and thighs (Hensinger et al., 1976). Symptoms are usually initiated or aggravated by strenuous activity, particularly by the repetitive flexion-extension activity of the spine common to oarsmen, gymnasts and divers, and are decreased by rest or limitation of activity (Hensinger et al., 1976; Micheli, 1979). A combination of these factors can be seen in weightlifting with too much weight used in the military press, with incorrect technique in gymnasts, and with too rapid advances in running or swimming.

Physical examination often demonstrates some tenderness in the region of the low back. There can be some splinting or guarding with restriction of side to side motion, particularly if the condition is of acute onset. Hamstring tightness is commonly found in the symptomatic patient (80%) (Hensinger et al., 1976; Turner and Bianco, 1971). If tightness of the hamstrings is present, there will be marked restriction of flexion of the hips. Distortion of the pelvis and trunk with grossly abnormal gait can be clinically apparent in the more severe stages of spondylolisthesis but is seldom found in the child with spondylolysis or Grade I spondylolisthesis.

Children, unlike adults, seldom have objective signs of nerve root compression such as motor weakness, reflex change, or sensory deficit and rarely

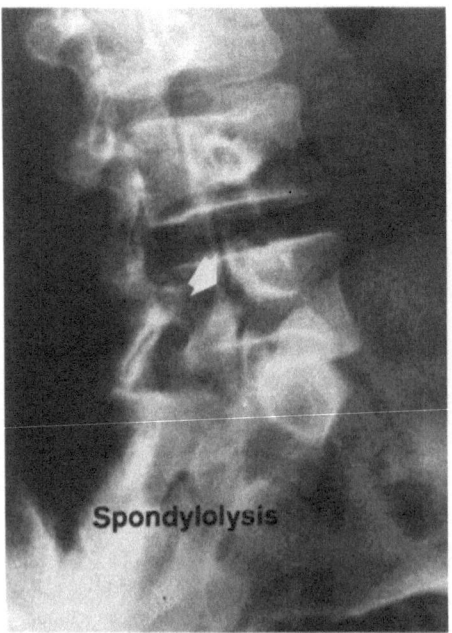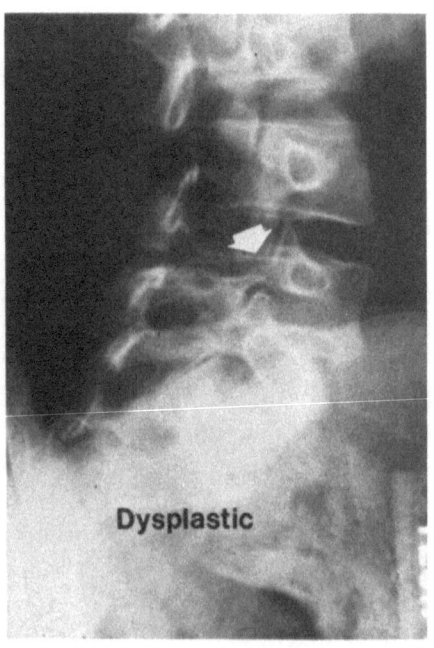

a   b

Fig. 7. a Oblique view of the typical spondylolysis or break in the pars interarticularis (arrow) seen with the isthmic form (type II). **b** The dysplastic form (type I), demonstrating elongation and attenuation of the pars interarticularis

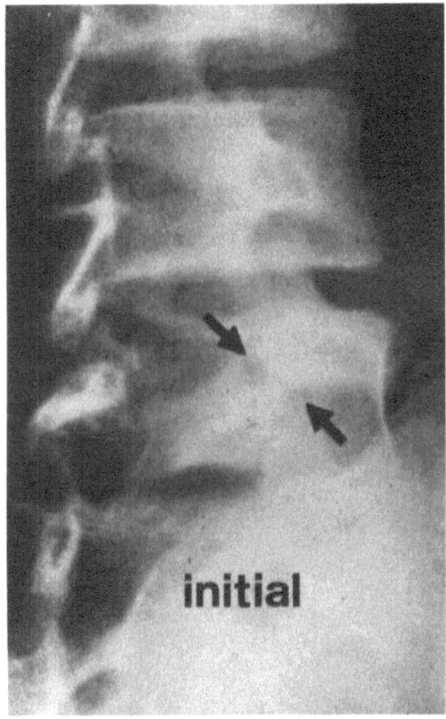 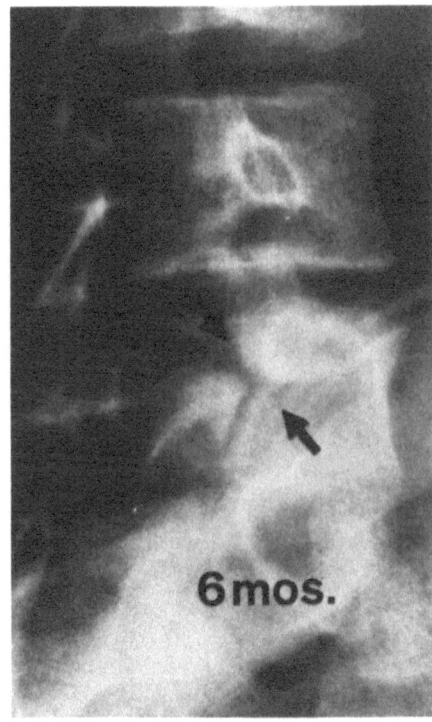

a   b

Fig. 8. Thirteen year old who felt a snap and sudden onset of pain in the low back during a swimming racing turn. **a** Oblique views demonstrate early spondylolysis (arrows) in the pars interarticularis. The narrow, irregular appearance suggests a recent injury. **b** Six months later, widening of the gap despite conservative treatment with cast immobilization. Patient had recurrence of pain due to fracture of the opposite pars interarticularis

have an associated disc protrusion (Hensinger et al., 1976; Turner and Bianco, 1971). The examination, however, must include a careful search for sacral anesthesia and bladder dysfunction since those findings require immediate attention.

If the radiolucent defect in the pars interarticularis (the spondylolysis) is large, it can be seen on nearly all roentgenographic views of the lumbar spine. If unilateral, as occurs in 20 percent of patients (Wiltse, 1961), and when not accompanied by spondylolisthesis, it can be a very subtle finding requiring special roentgenographic views. Oblique views of the lumbar spine are often necessary to view this area in relief and apart from overlying bony elements (Fig. 7). The "scotty dog" appearance of Lachapele with the defect appearing at the terrier's neck is a helpful visual aid to those inexperienced to the oblique roentgenogram (Fig. 7a). In an acute injury the gap is narrow with irregular edges, whereas in the longstanding lesion, the edges are smooth and

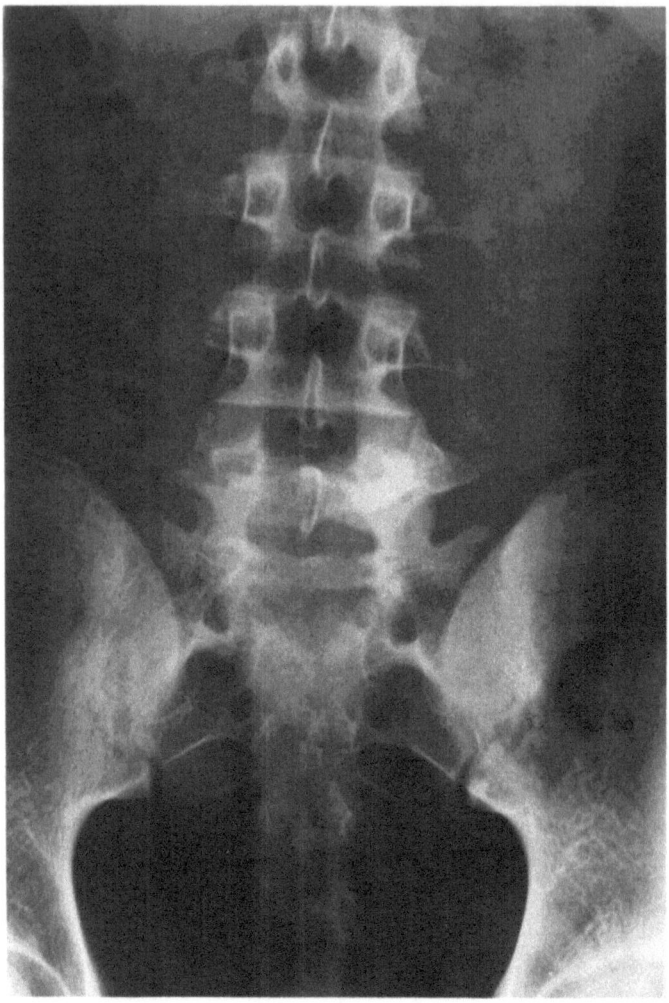

a

Fig. 9. Fifteen year old with low back pain. **a** Anteroposterior roentgenogram demonstrates reactive sclerosis and hypertrophy of one pedicle and lamina and contralateral spondylolysis of same vertebral segment. **b** Oblique roentgenographic view, demonstrating break in pars interarticularis. **c** Opposite oblique view demonstrating reactive sclerosis, which is physiologic response to stress resulting from repeated trauma in presence of unstable neural arch. Radiologically this may be confused with reactive sclerosis associated with osteoid osteoma

rounded (Fig. 8a, b). Children who are highly suspect clinically but in whom spondylolysis cannot be confirmed radiologically, particularly those in the stress reaction stage prior to fracture, may be detected by a bone scan. A CT scan also demonstrates the lesion quite nicely in many patients.

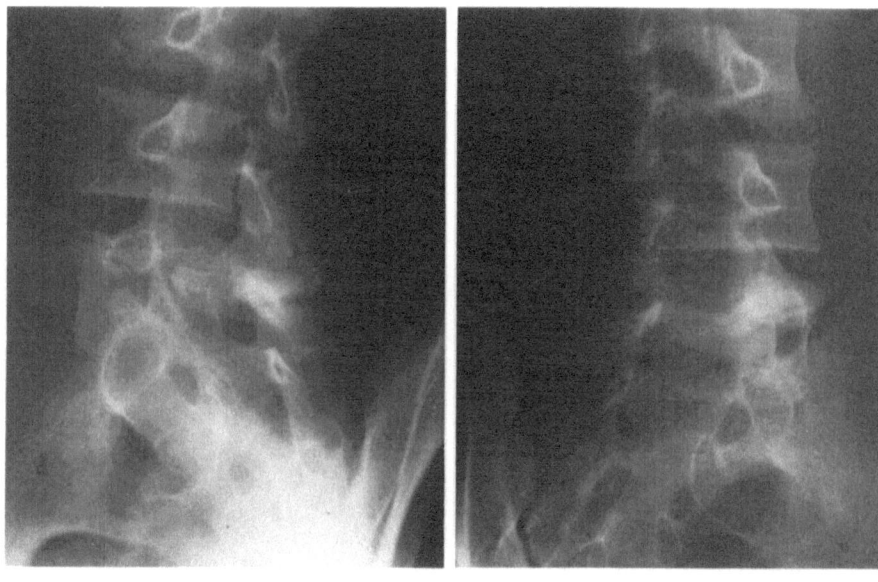

b   c

Less commonly children have poorly developed or anomalous posterior structures (dysplastic type), where the posterior facets appear to subluxate (Fig. 7 b). In children with the dysplastic type, rather than a gap or defect in the pars interarticularis, the pars can become attenuated like pulled taffy – the "greyhound" appearance of Hensinger (1976).

Sherman and associates (1979) described the unusual appearance of reactive sclerosis and hypertrophy of one pedicle and lamina and a contralateral spondylolysis in the same vertebral segment (Fig. 9 a–c). They suggested that this represents a physiologic response to stress, the result of repeated trauma in the presence of an unstable neural arch. Radiologically, this can be confused with the reactive sclerosis associated with an osteoid osteoma. This becomes an important concern since excision of a sclerotic pedicle in a patient with a contralateral spondylolysis can make the spine more unstable and lead to spondylolisthesis. The presence of a nidus should confirm the diagnosis of an osteoid osteoma, as discussed in Chap. 14. A bone scan will not be helpful in differentiating between the two, since both will exhibit an increased isotope uptake due to the presence of increased bone formation. One should be mindful that an osteoid osteoma typically causes pain at rest, often night pain and that pain is relieved by aspirin, and is persistent despite immobilization in a cast or brace. This is not characteristic of stress reactions which are generally relieved by rest or immobilization.

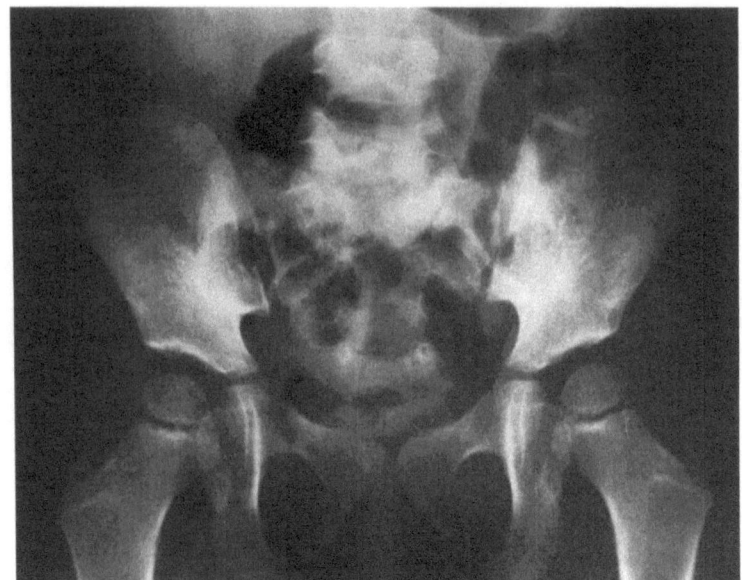

a

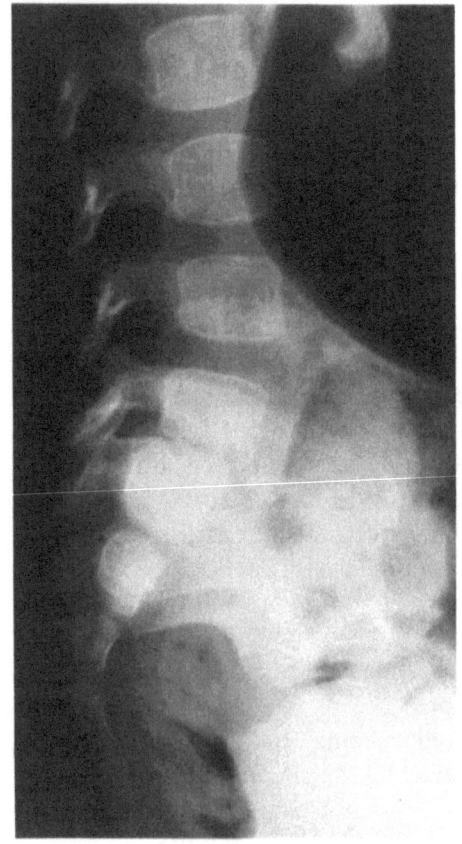

b

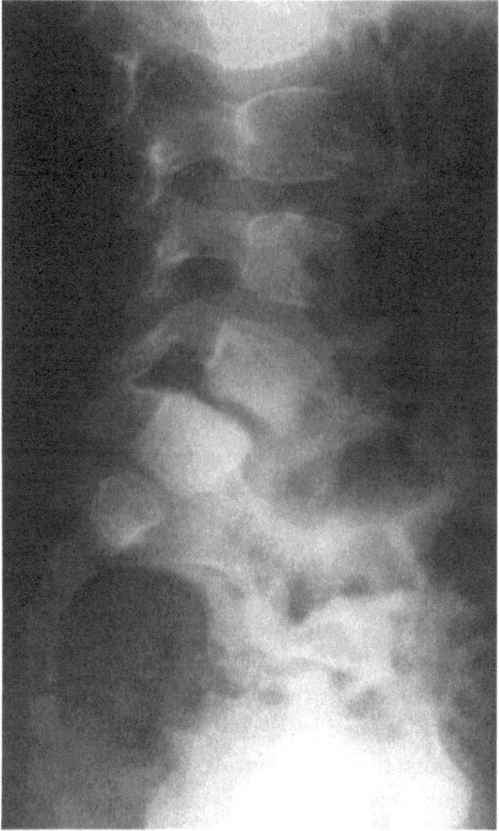

c

Fig. 10. a Anterior-posterior view of the L5-S1 of a three year old with discitis. **b** Note the narrowing of the disc space and endplate erosion. **c** Six months later the child is asymptomatic. There is partial reconstitution of the disc space but with a residual Grade I spondylolisthesis

Treatment of patients with spondylolysis/spondylolisthesis

Children and young adults have been reported to heal the spondylolytic defect after treatment with a cast or brace (Micheli, 1979). Typically the children have an acute onset of symptoms and the episode of injury can be clearly documented. Unfortunately, not all will heal with immobilization (Hensinger et al., 1976). However, immobilization should always be considered if the injury can be documented to be of recent origin. A bone scan may be helpful to indicate a continuing process versus one of long duration (Letts et al., 1986).

Children and teenagers in whom the spondylolysis has been present for a long time can be expected to respond to simple conservative measures (Hensinger et al., 1976). These include restriction of vigorous activities and back and abdominal strengthening exercises which are usually successful in controlling pain in children with mild backache and hamstring tightness. Patients with more severe or persistent complaints may require bedrest, immobilization in a cast or brace, and non-narcotic analgesics. Hamstring tightness is an excellent clinical guide to the success or failure of the treatment program. The majority of affected children have excellent relief of symptoms or only minimal discomfort on long-term follow-up (Turner and Bianco, 1971). A small percentage of young people with spondylolysis do not respond to conservative measures or are unwilling to curtail their activities, and may require surgical stabilization (fusion). Any child or adolescent discovered to have spondylolysis, especially those under 10 years of age, should be followed closely to detect progression. We do not advise those with asymptomatic spondylolysis or those with minimal symptoms to restrict their activities; about 7 percent of asymptomatic young men (18 to 30 years) in the U.S. have a pars defect and relatively few have persistent symptoms. Thus, limitation of activity in a growing child does not seem justified. It must be emphasized that it is quite uncommon for spondylolysis to be symptomatic in adolescence, and that the physician should resist the temptation to ascribe spondylolysis as the cause of symptoms in a symptomatic child. Rather, one should vigorously explore other possible causes of back pain. One should be particularly wary of the child whose symptoms do not respond to bedrest or who has objective neurologica findings.

Considerable information has been accumulated about the child with symptomatic spondylolisthesis, and thus results of treatment and prognosis are more predictable. Conservative measures are unsuccessful in controlling symptoms or postural deformity in over one-half of children, particularly when they present with Grades III and IV, spondylolisthesis. The majority of these children will require surgical intervention, and therefore should see an orthopedic surgeon (Hensinger et al., 1976). All patients should have a period of hospitalization and enforced bedrest prior to surgery to determine its necessity. Immobilization in a lightweight plaster or plastic jacket has been a helpful adjuvant in the preoperative evaluation (Hensinger et al., 1976). If conservative measures fail and surgery is indicated, a bilateral-lateral fusion is preferred (Chap. 3). Laminectomy is seldom indicated due to the low incidence of associated herniated nucleus pulposus and nerve root impingement (Turner and Bianco 1971). In general, if the patient's symptoms are related to activity and improved or resolved with bedrest or immobilization in a cast or brace, stabilization of the spine alone will achieve excellent long-term remission of symptoms (Hensinger et al., 1976). If symptoms or clinical findings persist despite bedrest and/or immobilization, or if the patient has difficulty with neurologic control of bowel or bladder, then one should obtain a myelographic examination and, if positive, an exploration of the spinal canal and decompression is recommended. Reduction of the spondylolisthesis is controversial and will not be discussed further in this text. Our preference is not to do so.

Disc herniation

Although it is not as common as in the adult, disc herniation can occur in children, with similar signs and symptoms (Bradford and Garcia, 1969; DeOrio and Bianco, 1982; Epstein et al., 1984; Garrido et al., 1978; Kumhana and Kalaoka, 1980) (Fig. 11 a, b). The onset of symptoms is usually less dramatic in children, and not as frequently associated with a physical incident (36%). DeOrio and Bianco (1982) suggest that disc herniation in children is more likely related to cumulative trauma than to a single event,

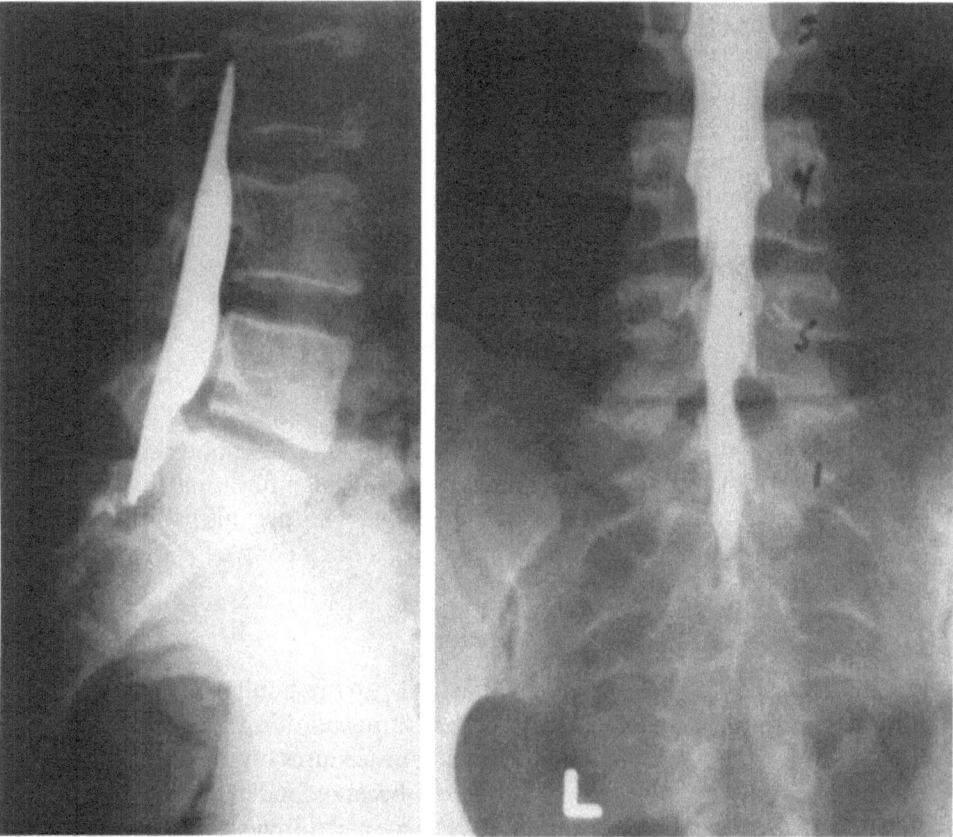

a   b

Fig. 11. Sixteen year old with a herniated nucleus pulposus. Myelogram demonstrates the lesion. **a** AP and **b** lateral

i.e. the result of a fatigue failure of the annular fibers. In the adolescent, back pain is a predominant finding and symptoms are typically increased with activity and relieved by recumbency. Coughing and sneezing may increase the pain. Local tenderness is inconsistent. A high percentage have positive straight leg raising and other sciatic nerve tension signs (Chap. 9). Muscle spasm is common and often causes splinting, scoliosis, and gait disturbances, but there are seldom objective neurologic findings. As in the adult, the L4-5 and L5-S1 levels are by far the most common. Plain film roentgenograms are typically normal in appearance. As in adults, the diagnosis will frequently require CT, MRI or myelographic confirmation.

Treatment of adolescent discal hernias

While there are similarities the adolescent disc hernia differs in both the clinical aspects and treatment from the adult variety of the same disease. The younger patients do not respond well to conservative care; and, thus, a far greater percentage will require surgical treatment than in adults. In adults the primary indication for surgical treatment is unresolved radicular symptoms. In children, radicular symptoms are seldom present and yet the disc hernias are often large. Surgical treatment can be expected to relieve the lower back pain, stiffness and hamstring spasm in the majority of patients (Bradford et al., 1974).

Spinal infection in children

Osteomyelitis

Spinal osteomyelitis occurs in both children and adults. In young children the process tends to be more often acutely septic with high fever and significant bone destruction, than is typical in the adult. The organism most often responsible for the infection is *S. aureus* as it is in osteomyelitis of the long bones (see Chap. 15).

Discitis

Discitis is a special case of spinal infection. In the adult spinal infection confined to the disc space is due to direct innoculation of the disc either during open surgery or percutaneous needle procedures on the disc. Primary discitis is almost non-existent in the adult because under normal circumstances the disc lacks a blood supply. However, in children vessels do traverse the disc thus providing a means of entrance for an organism. In both children and adults confirmation of a bacterial origin for "discitis" has been difficult to obtain (Boston et al., 1975; Menelaus, 1964; Spiegel et al., 1972). Nonetheless, this should be considered an inflammatory process which is secondary to infection because:

1. It ceases to exist after closure of the vessels (except by innoculation).

2. Experimental discitis which is pathologically and radiographically indistinguishable from clinical discitis can be produced by innoculation of only a few viable organisms which are not recoverable after 3 months (see Chap. 15).

3. The clinical syndrome is typical of infection.

4. Cultures have been obtained from the disc and a paravertebral abscess has been a complication of discitis in children.

Typically, when discitis occurs in childhood, there is an abrupt onset, accompanied by systemic signs of sepsis, fever and an elevated sedimentation rate. Often there is a history of a recent febrile illness, such as a sore throat or earache (Wenger et al., 1978). Widespread paravertebral muscle spasm and limited back motion are characteristic signs. The young child (less than 3 years) may refuse to walk. The pain is typically localized to the lumbar spine and can be quite severe with significant postural deformity and functional scoliosis. Depending on the level of involvement, there may be radicular pain to the abdomen, anterior thigh, and one or both lower extremities. Discitis is often confused with a variety of acute childhood illnesses, such as appendicitis, psoas abscess, and pyarthritis of the hip. Initially, the plain films of the spine may appear normal and the process can be difficult to diagnose. The bone scan has proven to be an accurate, rapid and safe method for diagnosis and localization (Wenger et al., 1978). Once localized, tomographic views will usually confirm the early endplate erosion and disc space narrowing which accompanies the onset of symptoms (Doyle, 1960). MRI is another sensitive method. However, it is not readily available and its cost-benefit value is questionable at this time. If associated with a high fever and signs of sepsis, aspiration of the disc space and blood cultures may be required. Surgical exploration to obtain a positive culture is rarely indicated (Wenger et al., 1978).

Slipped vertebral apophysis

This is a condition unique to teenagers, usually males, and generally associated with heavy lifting. Typically the posterior inferior apophysis of L4 (less commonly of L3 or L5) with its adjacent disc is displaced into the vertebral canal (Handel et al., 1979; Keller, 1974; Lippitt, 1976; Lowrey, 1973; Techakapuch, 1981). The injury is analogous to an acute slipped capital femoral epiphysis and occurs in the same age group. Slipped vertebral apophysis usually follows a traumatic incident, and may be precipitated by strenuous activity such as weightlifting, gymnastics or shoveling. Commonly,

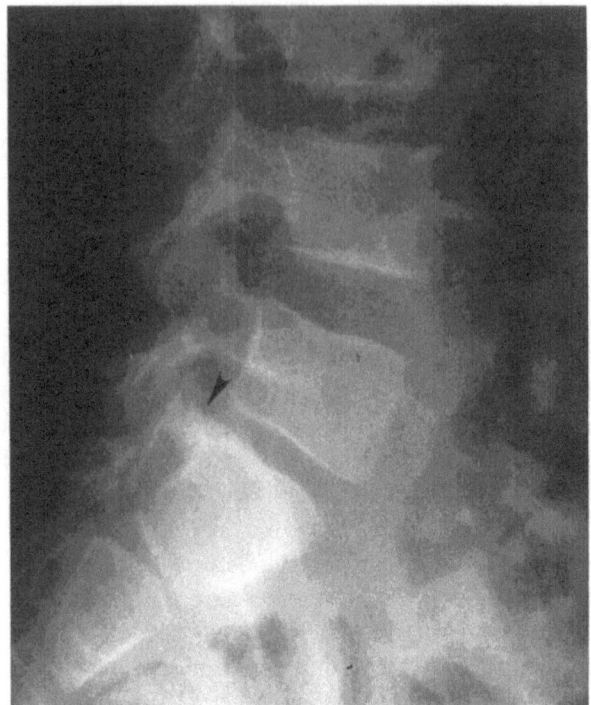

a

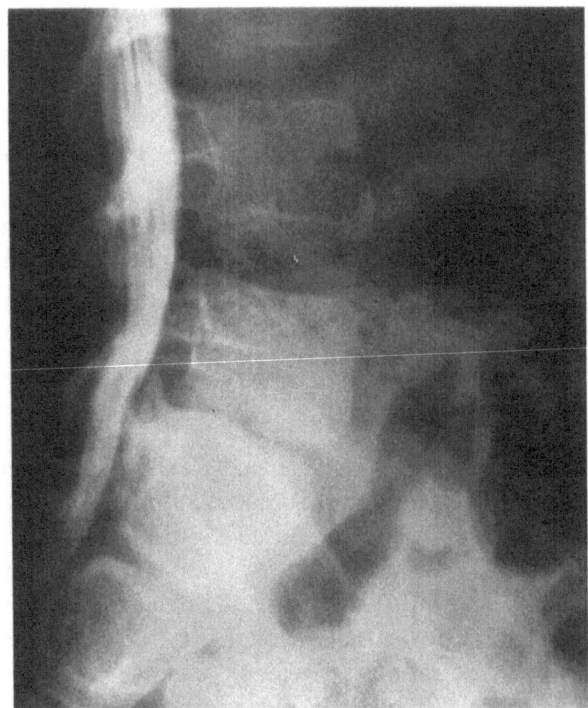

b

the children have signs and symptoms similar to those of an acute herniated disc. Neurologic findings such as muscle weakness and absent reflexes are often present. Roentgenographically, all cases demonstrate a small bony fragment (edge of the vertebral endplate) within the spinal canal. The myelographic appearance of the bony ridge (ring apophysis) and its adjacent disc is that of a large anterior extra-dural impression or complete block (Fig. 12a, b). Thus the condition is often confused with a herniated disc.

Treatment of slipped vertebral apophysis

Simple excision of the extruding disc seldom resolves the problem, rather decompression should include surgical removal of both the extruding disc and the bony ridge, which usually results in excellent relief of symptoms.

Disc space calcification

This is a rare clinical syndrome of uncertain etiology which usually involves the cervical spine, but can occur in the thoracic and lumbar region (Meinick and Silverman, 1963; Schechter et al., 1972; Sonnabend et al., 1982). Boys are affected twice as often as girls, commonly around seven years of age. The child presents with pain, stiffness, and local tenderness. There may be signs of inflammation with an elevated temperature, increased sedimentation rate and leukocytosis. The condition responds quickly to symptomatic treatment. Occasionally, the involved disc is weakened by the process and can herniate into the spinal canal (McCartee et al., 1972; Peck, 1957).

Juvenile ankylosing spondylitis (JAS)

This seronegative arthropathy is usually a disease of young adults, but can begin in males as young as six years of age. It has been estimated that 1 of 1000 boys under seventeen develop ankylosing spondylitis (Cassidy, 1982). In retrospective reviews 8.6 percent of patients with seronegative spondylarthropies had spinal complaints as teenagers, usually with onset between 10–15 years (Hart, 1955; Schaller, 1977). However, there is a considerable

---

Fig. 12. Slipped vertebral apophysis at L5 in a thirteen year old. **a** Note the small flake of bone (arrow), and **b** appearance of the myelogram which could be confused with a herniated disc. (Reproduced with permission from Callahan DJ et al. (1986) Intervertebral disc impingement syndrome in a child. Spine 11: 402–404, Harper and Row, Philadelphia)

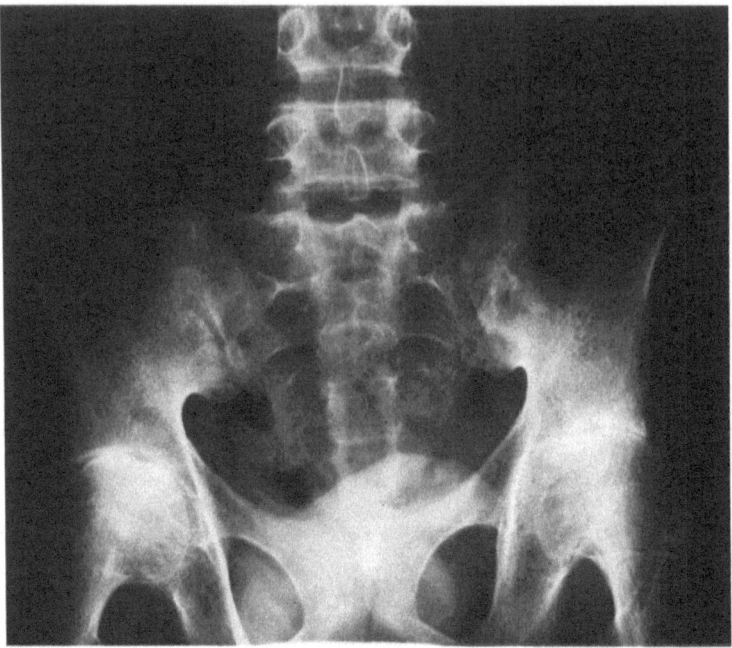

Fig. 13. Sacroiliac joint changes in a sixteen year old with rheumatoid spondylolysis

delay before the diagnosis is finally established. In 24 percent, the presenting complaints are related to the axial skeleton with morning stiffness and pain in the region of the SI joints (Kleinman et al., 1977). Approximately half the patients develop a transient arthritis of the larger peripheral joints. Common features include asymmetrical involvement of the joints, exacerbation of the pain at night, decreased chest expansion, a predilection for males, and a significant familial incidence. Routine laboratory studies are nonspecific, but 90 percent of white patients with juvenile ankylosing spondylitis will have the HLA-B27 antigen. Unfortunately, roentgenographic findings are rare during the early course of the disease. Although involvement of the SI joints appears first (Fig. 13), and is necessary for the diagnosis of ankylosing spondylitis, it can take 3–4 years before it can be seen roentgenographically (Kleinman et al., 1977). Radionucleid studies are often positive before roentgenographic findings occur, and CT scanning of the SI joints has been shown to be quite helpful in establishing the diagnosis early.

Benign neoplasms

Eosinophilic granuloma

A localized compression fracture without history of trauma or following a trivial injury should suggest the possibility of eosinophilic granuloma of the vertebra. Most of the children are between 2 to 6 and pain is seldom severe (Nesbit et al., 1969). Commonly there is a complete collapse of the body (vertebra plana), seldom the lytic appearance that is more commonly associated with involvement of the skeleton in other areas. Several vertebral bodies may be involved, in one study as many as eleven (Nesbit et al., 1969). The intervertebral disc is not involved and its thickness is retained. Unlike an infectious process, such as tuberculosis, a paravertebral soft tissue mass is uncommon. The prognosis is good for spontaneous resolution in the majority of children, with some growth in height of the vertebral body. But, complete restitution seldom occurs.

Osteoid osteoma/osteoblastoma

The most common bone forming tumors in the spine are the osteoid osteoma and osteoblastoma (Keim and Reina, 1975; Kirwan et al., 1984; Mehta and Murray, 1977; Schaller, 1977). Pain and scoliosis are nearly universal in children with these tumors (Fig. 2). Symptoms commonly occur at night (83%) and are usually aggravated by activity. Radicular pain can occur with marked spinal stiffness (89%). Osteoid osteoma can be very reactive, or very small, and hard to find on the initial radiographs, leading to prolonged delay in diagnosis. Thus a bone scan and computerized tomography are very helpful, both for localization and diagnosis (Fig. 2). The site of the lesion usually corresponds closely to the apex of the curve on its concave side. Osteoblastoma resembles osteoid osteoma in having a highly vascular matrix with much osteoid tissue, but is usually much larger and thus more easily discovered (Kirwan et al., 1984). They expand and destroy the involved bone but are surrounded by a shell of cortical new bone.

Aneurysmal bone cyst

Aneurysmal bone cysts are particularly common in the sacrum, but can occur in any area of the spine (Fig. 14a, b). They usually attain very large size before weakening the bone sufficiently to precipitate symptoms.

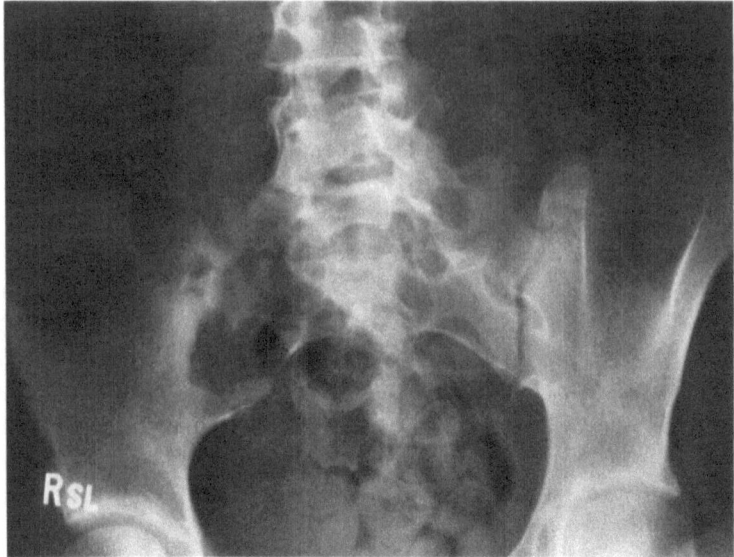

a

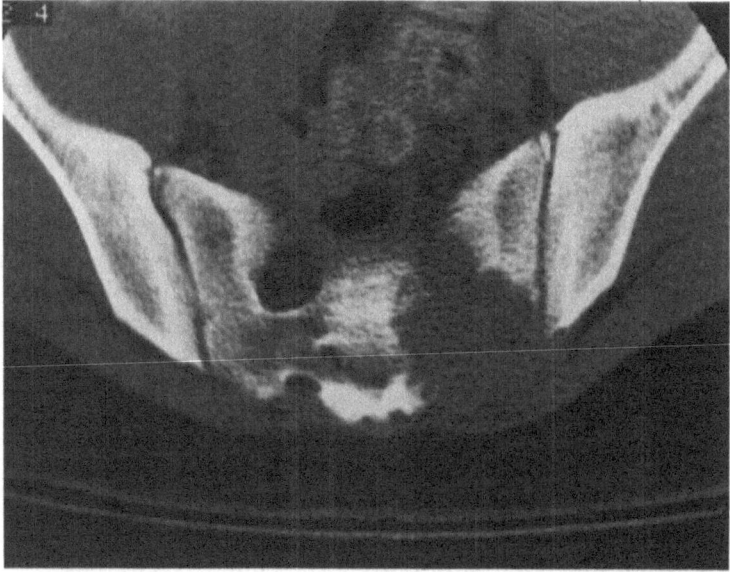

b

Fig. 14. Aneurysmal bone cyst of the sacrum in a fourteen year old. **a** Anterior-posterior roentgenogram of the pelvis. Overlying gas shadows and fecal material in the bowel prevent an adequate examination of the sacrum. **b** CT scan reveals a large aneurysmal bone cyst

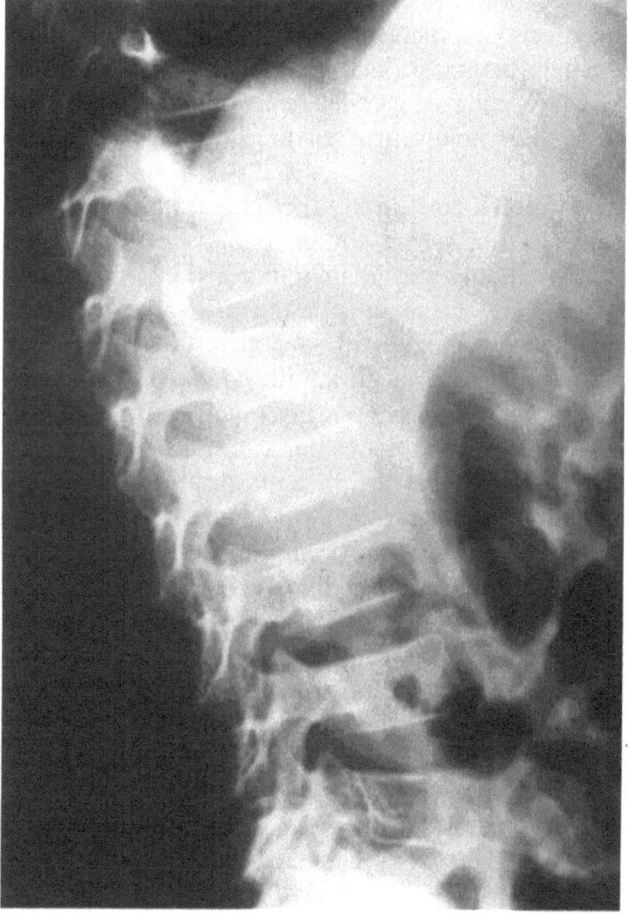

Fig. 15. Four year old with acute lymphatic leukemia demonstrating multiple compression fractures of the lumbar spine and no history of injury. Presenting symptoms were that of back pain. Initially child abuse was erroneously suspected

Malignant neoplasms

Primary malignant tumors in the spine are rare in children, the most common being Ewing's sarcoma (Young and Miller, 1975). More often the malignancy is metastatic, and the majority are secondary to primary tumors of bone or bone marrow, such as osteogenic sarcoma, Ewing's sarcoma, leukemia (Fig. 15), and Hodgkin's (Fernbach et al., 1977; Leeson and Makley, 1985; Young and Miller, 1975). Displacement of the normal bone forming elements by the abnormal cells can make the vertebra structurally weak, so that it collapses with minor trauma (Ogden and Ogden, 1982) (Fig. 15). Back pain is a common initial complaint, usually localized to the area of the collapse.

Neurologic complications are rare. The bone scan is the most sensitive method for early diagnosis of a metastasis or primary bone tumor, and in many children is more helpful than skeletal surveys (Gilday et al., 1977; Leeson and Makley, 1985). Many children with leukemia or lymphoma will have visceral involvement as well as involvement of the skeleton at other sites than the spine.

In children, skeletal metastases to the spine from other sources are most commonly from neuroblastoma and rhabdomyosarcoma, less often from teratoma, teratocarcinoma and Wilm's tumor (Leeson and Makley, 1985; Young and Miller, 1975). Depending on the series reported, up to 70 percent of patients with neuroblastoma will have metastatic skeletal disease at the time of their initial diagnosis or during the course of their treatment (Fernbach et al., 1977). The spine is typically involved with diffuse permeative destruction of bone similar to the changes seen in the metaphyseal areas of long bones with cortical destruction and variable amounts of periosteal reaction. Rhabdomyosarcoma is the most common soft tissue malignancy in children, and spine metastases occur in 30–50 percent of patients (Maroteaux, 1979). Lesions are usually lytic or radiolucent but may also be blastic or mixed, and bony destruction is common. Metastatic skeletal involvement is more common in the younger child. In Leeson and Makley's (1985) review, 27 of their 39 patients with skeletal metastases were 7 years of age or younger. In their series the most common fracture was compression fracture of a vertebra, half of whom had spinal cord compression.

Summary

The vast majority of children with back pain will have unspecific problems that can be managed by simple methods. However, a few will have serious underlying problems that demand immediate attention. Not all will be apparent on the initial evaluation, but usually with a careful history, physical examination, and stepwise evaluation using plain films, bone scan, and occasionally more detailed studies, the problem can be identified and brought to a successful conclusion.

13 The patient with functional disease/malingering

Introduction

The problem of the perception of pain, the patient's potential advantages in having others perceive him as being the "victim" of a painful condition, and the inability of the physician to validly measure pain cause most examining physicians to delay the proper diagnosis of "psychogenic pain" and/or "central pain" to the potential detriment of all concerned. The detriment comes from the repetitive and redundant search for a nonexistent somatic cause for the pain and the institution of different unsuccessful treatments. In order for the physician to clearly understand the problem of functional disease and/or malingering it is essential to understand some basic modern concepts of pain, it is transmission, perception, and clinical presentation. In general, this was discussed in Chap. 1, and should be reviewed before reading further into this chapter.

Misconceptions about pain

The simplistic notion of pain as "just another sensation" is the greatest stumbling block to the understanding of the patient with chronic pain complaint. The concept of pain as a sensation like vision, hearing, tasting, etc. does not explain either the process of the perception of pain or anything about how it is communicated to others. The inadequate and incomplete concept that "pain" is appreciated by a "receptor", transmitted by an afferent nerve to a spinal tract to the thalamus, and then to a "pain area" in the cerebral cortex does not explain many aspects of either acute pain, chronic pain, or the much more difficult exaggerated (functional, psychogenic, conversion hysteria, malingering, etc.) pain complaint.

Fallacy 1: Pain has a specific receptor

It appears that some free nerve endings (nociceptors) respond only to levels of stimulation which approach the intensity sufficient to result in tissue injury. It is also true that excessive stimulation of any receptor may be perceived as painful. Conversely, tissue injury can occur without the perception of pain.

Fallacy 2: Pain is a sensation like vision, etc.

Pain is a much more complex sensation than that of seeing, smelling or touching. There is no single center in the cerebral cortex for the perception of pain, but rather it is an integrated function of several areas of the cerebral cortex. Many aspects of pain are more like an emotion than a sensation. Many patients will describe their pain experience in emotive terms such as torturing or grueling rather than with terms which describe a bodily state such as cramping, aching or burning. Emotional and other psychological factors will modify pain. This modification may be either toward diminishing the pain or accentuating it. The well-known example of the soldier or athlete ignoring a major injury until the end of the battle, reflects the potential for complete inhibition of pain; while the opposite extreme of severe disabling pain complaint in the absence of any tissue injury is also a common experience.

Fallacy 3: "You can see that he/she is in pain"

The person suffering from pain is the sole source of information about that experience. Their pain is entirely subjective, personal, and private. There is no way that an outside observer is able to validate the statement "I am in pain". Pain behavior such as writhing or grimacing are statements about pain, but not "pain" per se.

Fallacy 4: Pain is quantifiable

Just as pain is a subjective experience, the only measure of the intensity of a person's pain experience is his/her personal statement as to the intensity of the pain. Furthermore, the perception of pain is dependent upon the state of consciousness and even the presence of a distraction can alter or eliminate the pain. Many patients do volunteer that they do not have pain during working hours, but suffer at night.

Fallacy 5: Pain is a universal phenomena that is the same for everyone

Different cultures view pain behavior differently. Some cultures appear to disapprove of the expression of pain and punish pain behavior while rewarding the tolerance of noxious stimuli, as did the plains Indians in America. Other cultures reward pain behavior and appear to approve the loud public display of agony even to the point of vesting the "pain" with religious importance.

Fallacy 6: The physical stimulation of a nerve is required for the perception of pain

Most reports of pain by a patient to a physician are undoubtedly due to the stimulation of nerve endings by some noxious stimuli; however, pain can be induced by other means such as suggestions (hypnosis). "Phantom limb pain" is pain perceived as originating in the missing limb following amputation. It occurs in the absence of afferent impulses and is not due to stimulation of neuromas in the stump.

Chronic neurogenic pain

There are three general types of chronic neurogenic pain based on its origin: (1) central; (2) spinal cord; and (3) peripheral (Table 1). Central neurogenic pain may occur following stroke or as a complication of chronic demyelinating diseases such as multiple sclerosis. A spinal cord mechanism for the production of chronic pain probably also exists. Animal studies following multiple dorsal rizotomies, and human experience in instances of traumatic dorsal root avulsion, suggest that the result of this type of deafferentation can lead to chronic pain input from the cord itself. The peripheral chronic neurogenic pain syndromes are collectively called "causalgias" and are well known and well described elsewhere. Psychogenic factors are almost always important in these neurogenic pain syndromes, and adjuvant psychologic treatment is usually necessary and important.

Table 1. Chronic (neurogenic) pain syndromes

No ongoing nociceptive stimulus
Possible central generators; e.g., post stroke
Possible cord generators; e.g., deafferentation
Possible peripheral generators; e.g., causalgia
Past mental health good – reactive depression

Depression

Patients who experience chronic pain frequently have an associated depression (Table 2). It has been hypothesized that there may be a chronic serotonin and/or endorphin abnormality which underlies both of these clinical entities. Recent clinical experience has demonstrated that tricyclic antidepressants may relieve chronic pain in some patients (Chap. 3). It has been postulated

Table 2. Depression

Loss of interest in self, work, family, and sex
Change in sleep pattern – usually sleeplessness
Morning headaches
Weight loss
Fearfulness
Irritable
Withdrawn
Tearful
Anxious or distracted

that these drugs have an effect on both endorphin and serotonin central nervous system mechanisms. Ward (1986) has demonstrated that the administration of fenfluramine which causes the release of serotonin can accurately predict those patients who would find relief from chronic pain through the use of tricyclic antidepressants. Ward further demonstrated that these agents did not influence the levels of central beta-endorphins.

Psychogenic pain

The distinction between conversion hysteria, hypochondriasis, malingering, and pain of somatic origin is essential when dealing with patients complaining of back pain. The tools that the physician has at his command are: the history as obtained from the patient; the history from a relative, friend or associate of the patient; the physical examination; outside observation of the patient's behavior; and psychological testing.

Conversion hysteria

Conversion hysteria is the transformation of an emotional conflict into a physical symptom (Table 3). The symptoms may be of a great variety, but for our purposes three are of greatest importance: paralysis, numbness, and

Table 3. Conversion hysteria

Primary gain
Little anxiety – La belle indifference
Over-dramatic presentation
Inconsistency – history and physical
Cooperative to the point of excess
Pleasant

pain. The patient's choice of symptoms is unconscious, and serves the purpose of fulfilling a need. The so-called "primary gain" is the degree to which this need is gratified by the hysterical symptom. In this regard, patients will demonstrate very little anxiety while relating the story to the examiner, and may even demonstrate *la belle indifference* more or less in proportion to the degree that the symptom satisfies the unconscious need or wish. The presentation is frequently over-dramatic in the language used and inconsistently presented. For example, the patient may be smiling while describing the current agonizing pain that he is experiencing. There is, frequently, the additional inconsistency of a weakness or numbness that does not follow anatomic or physiologic patterns.

Typically, the patient will be co-operative and allow unlimited testing, hospitalizations, and even painful surgeries. If the patient is seen for the first time many years after the initial onset of the symptoms the problems will be much more complex than originally. There may have been many treatments, the complications of which, may have resulted in significant physical disease which may be untreatable. The element of "secondary gain" eventually becomes a complicating factor in that the patient may now be receiving some form of compensation for the illness. The physician will find increasing resistance by the patient to any attempt to uncover the source of the symptoms.

Hypochondriasis

In distinction to conversion hysteria, the hypochondrial patient demonstrates severe concern for the most trivial symptom and worries endlessly that the symptom represents the most severe of diseases (Table 4). These patients never accept their symptoms with equanimity; but, rather, ricochet from physician to physician until they find someone who will "take me seriously".

Table 4. Hypochondriasis

Excessive worry about trivial symptoms
Anxious/frequent visits/frequent calls
Never satisfied
Forever seeking/multiple physicians
Few or no physical findings

Somatization disorder

One of the most difficult categories of patient is that of "somatization disorder". This is a chronic, disabling affliction which usually affects women beginning before the age of thirty years. It is characterized by the frequent

Table 5. Somatization disorder

Female
Begins before age thirty
Multiple somatic symptoms for which no reasonable cause is ever found
Recovery rare

---

complaint of multiple somatic symptoms for which no cause is found. These patients constitute between 0.2 and 2 percent of the adult female population, but utilize nearly ten times the value of health services used by the remainder of the population. They unnecessarily spend an average of more than seven days in the hospital each year per person. The recovery rate appears to be only 2 percent per year. Psychiatric care does not seem to improve the recovery rate, but it does reduce the over-all cost of care by about 50 percent.

Malingering

By "malingering" we mean that the patient is consciously attempting a deception for secondary gain which is usually some financial reward, although many other rewards are possible. The evidence, that malingering exists to a greater rather than lesser extent, is present, in the U.S. at least at every turn in the care of worker's compensation cases. Patients on workers' compensation consistently require longer to recover from the same illness than their non-compensated fellow sufferers. The compensation patients also consistently respond more poorly to any and all treatment modalities, but recover rapidly following a financial settlement. Prior to settlement the compensation patient tends to cooperate poorly with treatment.

It has been said repeatedly that it is quite difficult to distinguish the patient with conversion hysteria from the *conscious malingerer*. Here the first important distinction is "conscious". The malingerer needs to work every moment to maintain the charade, and thus will feel the need to let down his guard and relax when he feels that he is not being observed by those hostile to his cause. The conversion hysteric, on the other hand, is able to maintain the symptoms indefinitely; even to the point of developing joint contractures and other secondary physical changes. The malingerer, in contradistinction to the conversion hysteric, is usually noticeably hostile and nervous. He is resistant to testing, and will refuse treatment offered in good faith by the naive practitioner. Typically, the malingerer will miss multiple appointments and "forget" to bring records or radiographs when he does keep an appointment. Another ploy is to push the follow-up appointment far into the future so as to avoid the discovery that the once real illness has recovered. A common variation of malingering seen in workers' compensation is the exag-

Table 6. Malingering

Secondary gain
Conscious deception
Very slow or no recovery
Poor response to treatment with "worsening"
Hostile
Cooperates poorly with treatment
Cooperates poorly with testing/does not complete tests
Nervous
Late for visits
"Forgets" records
Spreads visits as far apart as possible/numerous cancellations
Abandons symptoms/signs when believed to be unobserved
Rapid recovery after financial settlement

Physical findings
Superficial/nonanatomic tenderness
Pain on axial loading
Pain on simulated rotation
Distraction tests positive
Nonanatomic weakness and/or numbness

---

geration and prolongation of a real injury's severity and duration of disability. Unfortunately, this is occasionally with the collusion of an unscrupulous fellow worker or an attorney. The most dangerous risk of this behavior is the possibility that the patient may have to accept dangerous treatment for a minor condition and end up with a complication which is far worse than the original complaint. Unfortunately, there are only two ways to diagnose the malingerer with any degree of certainty: (1) observe the patient abandon the symptom, or (2) elicit the patient's confession. Neither of these is as difficult as it may seem at first sight; patients may lose their limp on leaving the office or even solicit the complicity of the physician in their "innocent" fraud against the "rich insurer".

Inappropriate history and physical findings

In 1984, Waddell and coworkers published a now classical article on psychologic factors in patients with chronic low back pain. The study identified seven items of history which can be best described as "inappropriate descriptions of disease" and seven items that constitute "inappropriate responses to physical examination". Although they have been described in Chap. 2 they are so germain to this chapter that they will be repeated here.

Under normal circumstances, when a patient visits a physician, the description of his complaint can be expected to conform loosely to certain well recognized patterns of disease. Any patient's description may deviate to a greater or lesser extent from the text-book description of a known disease. If the patient's description deviates in major ways for the standard kinds of description of lumbar back pain (as presented in the previous chapters) then there are three possibilities to be considered: (1) a new disease is being described; (2) an old disease is being described with a new presentation; or (3) the patient's description represents a misrepresentation which is either conscious or unconscious. Items 1 and 2 are always possible, but are extremely rare. Item 3 is common enough in chronic low back pain that it can be said to constitute a 'disease of its own', which in our western industrial society, might be called "lumbar psychological distress syndrome". This may be over-generous in a number of instances when the patient is consciously attempting a deception (malingering).

Waddell identified twenty-two inappropriate symptoms which apply to lower back pathology. These were culled down to seven symptoms, which were quite rare in patients with identified spinal pathology but common in those without significant pathology. These seven symptoms are: (1) tail bone pain, (2) whole leg pain, (3) whole leg numbness, (4) whole leg giving away, (5) no pain-free spells, (6) intolerance of treatments, and (7) emergency admissions to hospital(s). These seven symptoms may occur at random in patients with identifiable lumbar spine pathology, but if as many as three are present in any one patient then there is a strong possibility of "lumbar psychologic distress syndrome".

The seven inappropriate physical findings function in much the same manner. They should be considered in the context of the whole patient's presentation and are of little significance singly. Waddell's seven inappropriate physical findings are: (1) superficial tenderness, (2) non-anatomic tenderness, (3) pain on axial loading, (4) pain on simulated rotation, (5) distraction straight leg raising, (6) regional weakness, and (7) over reaction. We have modified this list to include giving away or "ratchet weakness", Hoover's test, and non-dermatomal numbness. There are a few subtleties that the experienced examiner can add to this list. For instance, lumbar range of motion may be quite different when tested with the patient standing and sitting.

Psychological testing

A detailed analysis of the many testing instruments which have been adapted for the study of the "low back pain" patient or developed specifically for this purpose is beyond the scope of this chapter. The Minnesota Multiphasic Personality Inventory (MMPI) is perhaps the most widely used test for an attempt at evaluation of the psychologic status of the patient with low back-pain complaint. This test is cumbersome to administer, time consuming, expensive, and has limited application in the out patient care of the patient with a lumbar spine problem. Furthermore, there are significant questions as to the value of this test in the evaluation of patients with "psychologic pain complaint". The most direct criticism of this test is that it was not designed for the purpose of evaluation of the low back-pain patient. Also, for non-English speaking countries, and to some degree for English speaking countries outside the U.S., MMPI is less meaningful.

A pain "thermometer" or a visual analog scale is a device commonly used for the monitoring of the progress of a patient through treatment. This test is self-administered, easily understood, simple, reproducible, and may give some limited information with respect to the possibility of exaggeration of complaints.

The Million Behavioral Health Inventory is another test which was not specifically designed for the analysis of low back-pain patients but which appears to have some value in detecting those psychological factors which may worsen physical illness (Gatchel et al., 1986). As experience with this test grows its value in the evaluation of the low back-pain will be determined.

The McGill Pain Questionnaire (Melzack, 1975) and the Leavitt and Garron Low Back Pain Questionnaire (Leavitt and Garron, 1979) use individual words which the patient chooses to describe his pain problem. The Leavitt and Garron instrument has the advantage of having been specifically designed for the evaluation of the low back pain patient. This test is easily and quickly administered in the office setting, and has been found to be an accurate predictor of psychological disturbance in low back pain patients. It has also proven to be a reasonably accurate predictor of outcome of treatment in these patients (McNeill et al., 1986).

Deyo and Diehl (1986) have shown that three simple questions garnered in the history have predictive value in long term prognosis of patients with lower back pain complaints. Their patients were assigned one point if they reported that they "always felt sick", one point if they had had previous episodes of lower back pain, and one point if they had less than 9 years of formal education. The patients with 3 points said that their pain lasted an average of 41 days while those with 0 points had pain which lasted 12 days. All of the patients with 0 points were working at follow-up while only 50% of those with 3 points were employed at follow-up.

In patients in which there is felt to be the strong possibility of a significant psychological component to their experience of low back pain a complete battery of tests interpreted by a competent psychologist is recommended.

Summary

A patient's report of pain is private, personal and cannot be verified. Pain complaint may not be reflective of continuing tissue injury. Rather, the complaint of pain may be as the result of nervous system abnormality either peripheral, cord or central. Other pain complaints may come as a consequence of psychologic disturbance. These may include: depression, conversion hysteria, hypochondriasis, somatization disorder or malingering.

14 The patient with a spine tumor

Introduction

Tumors of the spine are comparatively uncommon, but the consequences can be disastrous. Therefore the possibility of a tumor in a patient presenting with low back pain should be kept in mind. Tumors producing lower back pain can be either benign or malignant; they can be either primary or metastatic; they can be in the bone, in the epidural space or inside the thecal sac. Primary tumors of the spine or its contents are rare, but metastatic tumors are not uncommon in older age groups. Metastatic lesions most often involve the bone, less often the epidural space, and rarely metastatic lesions may be intrathecal. On occasion, tumors involving the pelvis can mimic one of the lumbar spine syndromes, and tumors of the lower extremity can mimic sciatica (Boland et al., 1987; Mindell, 1981; Schajowicz, 1981; Sim et al., 1977; Simone and Lawner, 1982; Weinstein and McLain, 1987).

In many instances the tumor-induced symptoms do not allow accurate localization of the lesion on clinical grounds alone. Furthermore, the symptoms may not initially indicate that the cause of the patient's complaint are of a serious nature either to the physician or the patient. Long delays are often described between onset of symptoms and the eventual diagnosis and treatment. This delay is as often due to lack of concern on the part of the patient as it is due to confusion on the part of the physician (Mindell, 1981; Sim et al., 1977; Weinstein and McLain, 1977).

Both sexes and all age groups can be affected by spinal tumors. Primary tumors of the vertebral body are more often malignant than those of the posterior elements. Primary tumors of the spine are less likely to be malignant in young persons than in older adults. In a consecutive series from the University of Iowa the mean age of patients with primary malignancy of the spine was 49 years while the mean age for benign tumors was 21 years (Weinstein and McLain, 1987). Spinal tumors in older patients were most frequently found to be malignant, while benign neoplasms were rare. Conversely spinal lesions in children and adolescents were usually benign.

Figure 1 illustrates the common location of some of the tumors occurring in the vertebral column.

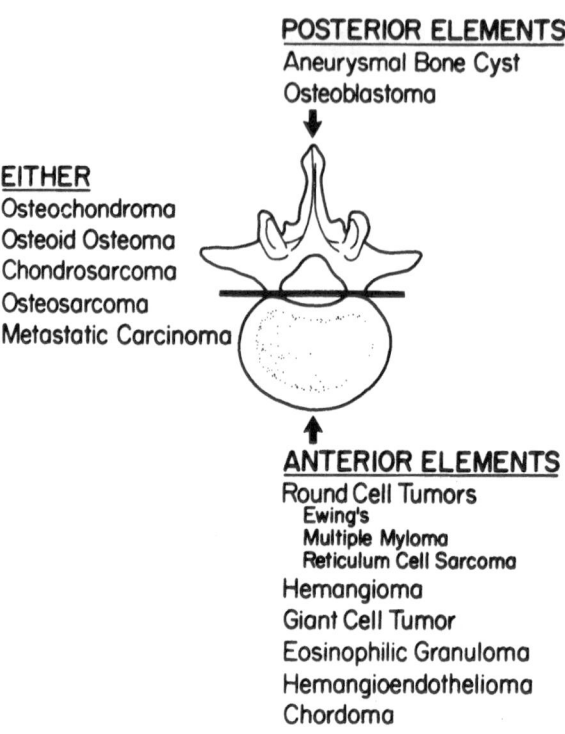

POSTERIOR ELEMENTS
Aneurysmal Bone Cyst
Osteoblastoma

EITHER
Osteochondroma
Osteoid Osteoma
Chondrosarcoma
Osteosarcoma
Metastatic Carcinoma

ANTERIOR ELEMENTS
Round Cell Tumors
   Ewing's
   Multiple Myloma
   Reticulum Cell Sarcoma
Hemangioma
Giant Cell Tumor
Eosinophilic Granuloma
Hemangioendothelioma
Chordoma

Fig. 1. Most frequent location of spine tumors

Signs and symptoms

Sim et al. (1977) have emphasized that signs and symptoms typical of a herniated intervertebral disc can be caused by primary tumors of the spine. The correspondence may actually be so great that the diagnosis is not suspected until the time of surgical exploration. Both benign and malignant tumors may masquerade as a disc herniation. Fortunately, in most instances the distinction can be made with relative ease. Night pain and night time sciatica should lead to suspicion of tumor. Severe pain unrelieved by rest suggests that the presenting complaint is not mechanical in origin, nor due to a benign nerve root compression. A gradual onset of perineal pain associated with constipation, rectal bleeding, or urinary dysfunction suggests a sacral tumor.

Spinal deformity along with pain may be the presenting complaint in patients with tumors (and also infection). In young persons the association of pain and scoliosis suggests the presence of an osteoid osteoma. The development of a kyphotic deformity in an adult suggests pathologic fracture (e.g., osteoporosis) or bone destruction due to tumor or infection.

Table 1. Signs and symtoms of patient with a spine tumor

Presenting complaints	Physical findingss
Unremitting back pain or little relief with rest	Local tenderness
Night pain or pain aggravated by lying down	Spasm or stiffness
Sciatica or sciatica at night only	Deformity
Perineal pain or numbness	Mass
Previous malignancy	
Deformity/scoliosis or kyphosis	*Radicular findings*
Weakness (in the extreme event – paraplegia)	Straight leg raising positive
Bowel or bladder disturbance	Reflex change
Mass	Weakness
Dramatic relief with ASA	Sensory change
(osteoid osteoma/osteoblastoma only)	
	Signs of cauda equina compression
General symptoms	Saddle anesthesia
Weight loss	Sphincter weakness
Fever	Detrusor weakness
Fatigue	Paraplegia

Both infections and tumors of the spine can present as severe and un-remitting low back pain and both may have an insidious onset. Furthermore, both tumors and infections may have concomitant signs and symptoms of radicular or cauda equina involvement.

The presence of low back pain in a patient with a previous history of malignancy must be considered to be due to metastatic disease until proved otherwise.

Benign tumors of the spine

Osteoid osteoma and osteoblastoma are variations of the same theme (Dahlin, 1978; Huvos, 1979; Schajowicz, 1981). The osteoid osteoma desig-nation, when used, indicates a lesion with a nidus smaller than 1 cm and with a surrounding sclerotic zone, while the osteoblastoma designation indicates a larger lesion without the reactive bone formation surrounding the nidus. From the clinical point of view it is valuable to consider these two lesions together. They are the most common benign lesions of the spine constituting fifty percent of all benign spinal tumors (Sim et al., 1977; Weinstein and McLain, 1987).

In young persons osteoid osteoma and osteoblastoma can be accompa-nied by a significant scoliotic deformity. This scoliosis will often resolve following successful removal of the lesion. However, when the patient is very young and the lesion is long standing, the curve can become structural and progressive (Keim and Reina, 1975; Kirwan et al., 1984; Ransford et al., 1984).

Osteoid osteomas and osteoblastomas are notorious for masquerading as herniated intervertebral discs when present in the lumbar spine. The tumor does not have to impinge upon a nerve to cause symptoms of pain in the sciatic distribution. Lesions of the lamina or pedicle can present with leg pain and even with a positive straight leg raising sign. The distinction to a disc problem can often be made on the basis of the presence of night pain and dramatic relief of pain with aspirin. Due to the decreasing use of ASA as a first choice in pain medication, an ASA test may have to be performed.

The diagnosis of osteoid osteoma/osteoblastoma can often be made of the plain X-ray studies of the spine. With the smaller lesions, bone scans and tomography (CT) are necessary to localize the lesion.

The treatment of osteoid osteoma/osteoblastoma is complete surgical excision. Failures of treatment are due to incomplete excision. We have found that an intraoperative bone scan is invaluable for both the localization of the lesion and for determining whether or not the entire lesion has been removed.

Other common benign bony tumors of the lumbar spine are: osteochondroma, giant cell tumor, hemangioma, and aneurysmal bone cyst. Chondromyxoid fibroma may also occur.

Benign intrathecal tumors involving the cauda equina are usually either neurofibromas or meningiomas (Simeone and Lawler, 1982). Gradually increasing symptoms of back pain or radicular pain may be present for a long period of time before they become sufficiently severe for the patient to seek medical help or for the physician to request appropriate tests. The meningiomas are more common in middle aged females while the neurofibromas are seen in a somewhat younger population. These lesions often cause night pain or pain on recumbency, but this is not invariable. Until very late in the illness the only complaint may be back pain. Myelography may be the only diagnostic possibility in these patients until very late in the disease process.

Primary malignant tumors of the spine

The signs and symptoms of the primary malignant tumors of the spine are not different from those of the benign tumors except, possibly in severity. The malignant lesions are more likely to present with neurological deficits (Weinstein and McLain, 1987). Many different primary malignant tumors of the spine exist. The most common are myeloma (plasmacytoma) and chordoma each constituting about twenty-five percent of the primary malignant tumors (Weinstein and McLain, 1987). Other primary malignant tumors include: osteosarcoma, chrondrosarcoma, fibrosarcoma, Ewing's tumor, lymphoma, and malignant giant cell tumor.

Chordoma, although common among the malignant primary spine tumors, is a relatively unusual tumor (4% of all primary bone tumors) with a predilection for the sacrum and occiput. Fifty percent of these tumors involve the sacrum and fifteen percent the vertebrae. The cell of origin is thought to be a notochordal remnant. The tumor occurs in any age group and is present in males twice as often as females. The tumor is usually slow growing in adults but can grow rapidly in children. When the tumor involves the sacrum the symptoms are those of local pain, perineal pain, perineal numbness, constipation, sexual difficulties, and urinary dysfunction. There is usually a presacral mass that is palpable on rectal exam. Finally, if left untreated, it results in a complete cauda equina syndrome (Mindell, 1981).

Chordomas are usually evident on plain X-rays but the full extent of the tumor may not be appreciated without CT examination. Calcifications may be present in the tumor mass and both osteolytic and osteoblastic bony lesions can be seen. In instances in which complete, wide excision of the lesion is possible a cure may be hoped for. However, most of these lesions are much too large to be resected when they are first found (Mindell, 1981).

Myeloma (plasmacytoma) can also present with symptoms of back pain and sciatica with radicular signs being an early symptom of the disease (Sim et al., 1977). Lesions greater than about 1 cm in diameter can be seen on plain X-rays as discrete punched out areas of bone, however, myeloma may also present as osteopenia. The sedimentation rate can be elevated in these lesions, and serum electrophoresis may reveal a monoclonal gamma spike. In myeloma the bone scan is not infrequently negative, especially in small lesions and lesions which do not cause a bony reaction (Boland et al., 1987). The existence of a true solitary plasmacytoma rather than an early stage of multiple myeloma is in doubt and reports including this lesion (plasmacytoma) should be viewed with skepticism (Simeone and Lawner, 1982). Chondrosarcomas are other comparatively common primary malignant spinal tumors (12% in Weinstein and McLain's study (1987)). They occur most often in patients past the age of 40, and are more frequent in men than in women. Growing comparatively slowly and metastasizing late, surgical removal of these tumors can sometimes be performed with a good result.

Osteosarcoma, Ewing's tumor, and lymphoma of the spine all have a poor prognosis; but survival statistics are improving yearly and so an aggressive treatment plan is warranted when these lesions are encountered (Russin et al., 1982; Shives et al., 1986; Weinstein and McLain, 1987).

Metastatic tumors of the spine

Breast, prostate, thyroid, kidney and lung tumors are commonly metastatic to bone and the spine is often involved in these metastatic deposits. About

60 percent of the metastatic neoplasms are in the spine. Treatment of these lesions is necessary for relief of pain, restoration of structural stability, and prevention of neurologic catastrophe. Aggressive surgical treatment is not likely to result in prolongation of life, but it may provide an improved quality of life for the time remaining. The majority of the metastatic lesions involve the vertebral body. Most of the lesions are osteolytic, but osteoblastic metastases also occur, particularly from prostatic carcinoma. As tumor destruction of the bone progresses the body of the vertebra collapses producing a kyphotic deformity with neural involvement by either direct extension of the tumor or mechanically due to severe instability leading to stretching, tearing or kinking of neural elements. Excision of a vertebral body and replacement with a methylmethacrylate, metal, and/or bone construct has a place in the management of these patients (Siegal et al., 1985). In the early stages metastatic tumors to the spine cannot be detected on plain films. A technetium bone scan is then helpful to rule out malignancy.

Diagnosis and treatment

Plain roentgenograms are the cornerstone of tumor diagnosis. They should be obtained in patients with persistent back pain and/or neurologic deficits. This is particularly true in children and elderly patients. When metastatic disease is suspected bone scans should also be obtained. Myelograms, myelogram/CT scans, and MRI are helpful in patients with neurological deficits. When identified, a thorough work-up should preceed biopsy or excision. This general work-up should include CBC, serum immunoelectrophoresis, lung X-rays, clinical examination of common sources of tumor, a bone scan and an intravenous pyelogram. This work-up and further treatment should be directed by a surgeon with an interest in orthopaedic oncology and/or spinal surgery.

15 The patient with spinal infection

Introduction

The key problem in spinal infection is the failure of the medical community to appreciate that these problems continue to exist and are actually relatively common and increasing in frequency. The increase in frequency is due to several factors: (1) Our elderly population is increasing, and even without concurrent illnesses this group has a less than normal competent immune system. (2) An increasing number of patients with immune deficiencies, either of the infectious acquired type or secondary to treatment of malignant or autoimmune disease. (3) Large migrations of populations from TB endemic regions.

In the past, the chief problems of spinal infections were those of tuberculosis; and, in the world community this disease remains the most important infectious disease of the spine (Medical Research Council, 1978, 1982). In a general medical or orthopaedic practice the incidence of haematogenous pyogenic infections has been quite low (Stauffer, 1975); however, iatrogenic infections are increasing in incidence as are opportunistic infections in immune incompetent patients. These infections are quite difficult to diagnose as they tend to be indolent and caused by organisms that were not considered to be pathogens in the past. In some of these infections, positive cultures may be difficult to obtain, especially if they have been present for a number of months. The difficult questions then become: (1) How does one know that the syndrome is assuredly caused by an infectious agent? (2) How does one choose the correct treatment if the organism is not identified?

Historical

Hippocrates and Galen (Major, 1948) both described spinal tuberculosis in great detail. Percival Pott of Guy's Hospital, London, described the paraplegia associated with spinal tuberculosis in the 18th century (Rang, 1966). It was not until the late 19th century that pyogenic infections of the spine were recognized as entities distinct from tuberculosis by Lannelongue (Steindler, 1929). Smith first described the discitis of childhood in 1933 (Table 1).

Table 1. Signs and symptoms suggestive of spinal infection

Acute	Chronic
Fever and chills	History in the past
Severe unremitting back pain	Weight loss
Radiation to groin, flank, or abdomen	History of TB, personal or family
Well localized spinal tenderness	member
Severe spasm	Night sweats
History of recent GU or GYN manipulation	Spinal deformity
History of recent spinal injection or surgery	Groin, thigh, or flank swelling
Immune deficiency	Origin from area with endemic TB
Exposure to unpasteurized milk	or fungal diseases

Tuberculosis and fungal infections of the spine

The incidence of spinal tuberculosis has been decreasing during the past century in Great Britain, western Europe, and the United States until the past several years (Hughes et al., 1986). The reversing trend is in part because of the recent development of a growing number of AIDS patients who, because of immune deficiency, are more susceptible to the development of infections including tuberculosis; and in part due to the increasing numbers of elderly. Further, there has also been a large migration of persons from endemic areas to regions which had not experienced a previously significant level of this disease; at least, not during this century (Table 2).

The sex ratio is equal, but the age incidence of spinal disease is quite different in differing ethnic groups. The Chinese in Hong Kong presenting with Pott's disease are usually preadolescent (Hodgson et al., 1960) while the Caucasian population in Great Britain are more often over age thirty-five.

Primary spinal fungal infections are rare (Morris, 1965; Winter, 1978; Eismont, 1983). In our experience they are seen in chronically ill patients, those receiving corticosteroids, patients with lymphomas or Hodgkin's disease, AIDS patients, and intravenous drug abusers. Patients receiving long term antibiotic therapy are also at risk, especially, from *Candida albicans*. Sporadically, coccidiodomycosis (Valley Fever), blastomycosis, and sporotri-

Table 2. Characteristics of spinal tuberculosis. Epidemiology

Ancient disease
In developing countries a disease of childhood
Western countries a disease of elderly and chronically ill
Steady decline in incidence for several hundred years until AIDS
One half of all bone and joint tuberculosis involves the spine

chosis have been observed in patients who are not members of the various groups with increased susceptability (Table 3).

It must be remembered that both tuberculosis and fungal infections are systemic diseases; and, thus, the spinal manifestations are only a part of the patients problem (Lifeso, 1985). The clinical presentation of either disease may be quite varied and may mimic many other diseases. There is fever, night sweats, malaise and weight loss as would be expected in a systemic disease. In addition, there will be the local findings of tenderness and muscle spasm, while deformity may also be present. Paraplegia may develop with progressive vertebral destruction and deformity, from pressure from an epidural abscess, and from direct involvement of neural elements (Hodgson et al., 1960).

The diagnosis of Pott's disease and of fungal infection of the spine depends first on the clinical realization that these diseases still exist in Western medical practice. Most physicians will practice for years without seeing either of these diseases, and this fact alone makes the diagnosis difficult. Further causes of difficulty in diagnosis are: symptoms may mimic other diseases; the disease develops slowly; radiographic changes may be late or absent; skin tests may be negative (14%); bone scan is negative in 35%; Gallium scan is negative in 70%; and neurologically impaired patients may have negative X-rays (Lifeso et al., 1985; Hughes et al., 1986) (Table 4).

The X-ray appearance of Pott's disease takes several patterns (Table 4). There may be central vertebral destruction, anterior scolloping, paravertebral abscess (Fig. 1 and Table 5), localized kyphosis, and destruction of

Table 3. Non-tubercular granulomatous infections of the spine. Fungal (rare)

Aspergillosis
Coccidiodomycosis
Blastomycosis
Cryptococcosis

Table 4. Clinical characteristics and diagnostic information on spinal tuberculosis

Now unusual
May mimic other diseases
Develops slowly
Radiographic changes may be late
TB skin tests (−) 14%
Bone scan (−) 35%
Gallium scan (−) 70%
Neurologic signs may occur without radiographic changes in bone

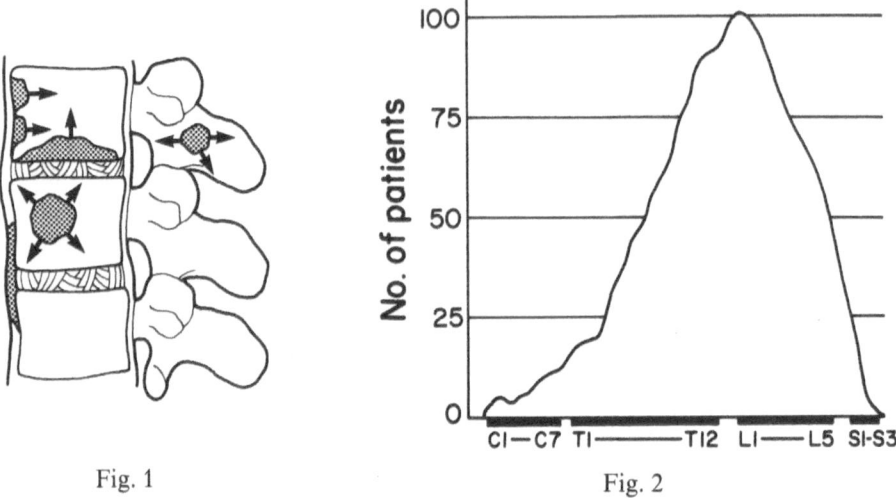

Fig. 1   Fig. 2

Fig. 1. Tuberculosis. Localization of foci within vertebra

Fig. 2. Tuberculosis. Relative involvement of the spine by levels

Table 5. Localization of tuberculous spinal foci

Under anterior longitudinal ligament	children
Anterior body	20%
Adjacent to end plate	60%
Arches	8%
Paravertebral abscess	commonly

adjacent vertebrae on either side of the intervening disc (Schmorl and Jung-hans, 1971). This may result in significant deformity (Table 6). There is also associated osteoporosis. TB most often involves the lower thoracic or upper lumbar vertebrae (Fig. 2). The diagnosis in these diseases is dependent upon tissue examination and culture; and, therefore, biopsy is essential. The culture and/or microscopic examination will be positive in more than seventy percent of the cases, but it is not universally diagnostic. Skin testing may be helpful in the diagnosis of tuberculosis. Neither skin testing nor serologic testing are helpful in blastomycosis, candidiasis, or sporotrichosis.

The treatment of tuberculosis or of fungal diseases of the spine requires that the physician address four different considerations: (1) the systemic nature of the disease, (2) the abscess and associated necrotic tissue, (3) the deformity, and (4) neurologic injury both actual and potential (Medical Research Council, 1978, 1982; Friedman, 1966).

Table 6. Spinal deformities in tuberculosis of the spine

Kyphosis
Scoliosis
Block vertebrae
Elongated vertebrae

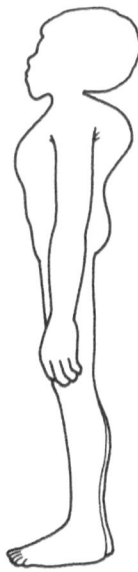

Fig. 3. Tuberculosis. Severe kyphosis

The systemic nature of the disease requires attention to adequate nutrition, exercise, and appropriate antibiotic therapy. Selection of the proper antibiotic requires positive identification of the organism and testing, in the case of tuberculosis, for sensitivities.

Tuberculous abscesses of any significant size require drainage, debridement of any associated necrotic tissue, and bone grafting of defects. Fungal abscesses should also be drained, but the safety of bone grafting in fungal diseases has not been established. Early deformity, in which rigid bony fusion has not occurred, can be corrected and maintained by bone grafting at the time that the abscess is drained. The eventual severity of the deformity is a function of the quantity of bone loss and, thus, is predictable to some extent. Late deformity (Fig. 3) does not require treatment unless the neural elements are being compromised. The gibbus deformity (sharply angled kyphosis) may cause myelopathy either as a result of direct pressure upon the cord or by vascular injury. The onset of myelopathy can be long after healing of the infectious focus. The surgical treatment of the late deformity can be quite complex and has a significant degree of risk. Therefore, anticipation and early treatment are preferred.

Vertebral osteomyelitis

There are three different categories of vertebral osteomyelitis: (1) pyogenic, haematogenous osteomyelitis, (2) discitis of childhood, and (3) iatrogenic discitis.

Pyogenic osteomyelitis is primarily a disease of adults and one half are older than fifty years (Stauffer, 1975) (Table 7). Now this is rarely a disease of children; however, Steindler (1929) describes it as primarily a disease of children. Today, children and infants most often acquire osteomyelitis of the long bones. When osteomyelitis of the spine does occur in children, it is a severe illness and should not be confused with the much more benign discitis of childhood (Eismont, 1982; Wegner, 1978).

Most osteomyelitis of the spine is the result of seeding from a distant site via a vascular route either via Batson's plexus or an arterial route (Wiley et al., 1959; Trueta, 1959; Batson, 1940).

Pyogenic, haematogenous osteomyelitis is not common but also not a rare disease and should be expected in any patient who presents with severe back pain which is unrelieved by rest (Stauffer, 1975). A spurious history of trauma is not unusual and may lead to delay in diagnosis. A recent history of urologic or gynecologic treatments and an elevated ESR should help to alert the physician to the possibility of osteomyelitis. On occasion an atypical presentation as abdominal pain, chest pain, or hip pain may confuse the issue (Kulowski, 1936; Puig-Gore, 1946). Constitutional symptoms such as fever may be absent, especially in the elderly. Again diagnosis at an early stage of the disease requires a sensitivity on the part of the physician to the possibly subtle differences in presentation of this disease from the more common causes of backache. If the possibility of vertebral osteomyelitis is not suspected the delay in diagnosis may be very long. In one series this delay was two months from the onset of symptoms (Griffiths, 1971). The history of a rather

Table 7. Epidemiology in pyogenic osteomyelitis of the spine

Adults–not often children
Uncommon
Blood borne
Following GU or GYN manipulation

Table 8. Bacteriology in pyogenic osteomyelitis of the spine

Staphylococcus aureus
Streptococci
E. coli
Anaerobes
Actinomyces
Brucella

gradual onset of the symptoms and the finding on physical examination of very well localized tenderness over the spinous process of the involved level are helpful clues, but are not specific for the diagnosis of vertebral osteomyelitis. Radicular symptoms may be present but, tend to be late, rather than early findings. The differential diagnoses must initially include fracture secondary to osteopenia, metastatic focus, and tuberculosis.

The most common organism is *Staphylococcus aureus* constituting about two thirds of the infections and *Enterobacteraciae* (e.g., *Serratiae, Protease,* and *Salmonellae,* and *Streptococci*) constituting most of the remainder. For the precise diagnosis and treatment it is essential that cultures be obtained. Occasionally, blood cultures in severely ill patients with clinical septicemia will be adequate; but the preferred practice is direct culture of the lesion, usually by needle aspiration (Table 8).

Radiographic findings are absent initially. After a week to ten days, vertebral destruction, frequently involving the endplate and adjacent disc becomes evident. There is usually an associated soft tissue swelling or paravertebral abscess. Massive destruction with significant deformity and sequestration are late findings. Vertebral osteomyelitis is frequently erroneously called "discitis" because of the involvement of the adjacent disc (Fig. 4). In

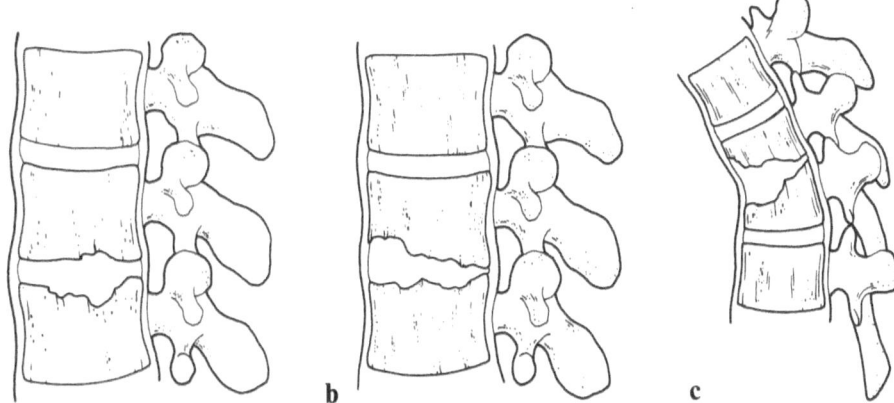

a   b   c

Fig. 4a–c. Pyogenic osteomyelitis. Progressive involvement of adjacent vertebrae leading to deformity

discitis, however, the disc involvement is primary, while in osteomyelitis the disc involvement is secondary. Initially, little may be seen on conventional X-rays. Magnetic resonance imaging, bone scanning, and conventional tomography are all useful in the early detection of vertebral osteomyelitis.

The treatment of vertebral osteomyelitis is three-fold: (1) proper antibiotic therapy, (2) adequate rest, and (3) timely surgical treatment. The proper antibiotic therapy is dependent upon adequate culture of the offending organism with sensitivities (Waldvogel, 1970, 1980). The duration of therapy should be at least six weeks with documented blood levels of the antibiotics. It is often necessary to give prolonged IV therapy using an implanted catheter with self administration of the drugs under the supervision of a visiting home nurse. Adequate rest may be different at different stages of the illness. Initially, bed rest may be required; while, later in the illness, an orthosis will be sufficient. A few of the patients will require surgical drainage of an abscess, decompression of neural elements, and correction of deformity with spinal fusion.

Discitis

De novo disc space infections are almost exclusively a childhood disease. The small vascular branches which penetrate the end plate pores and enter the disc cartilage are not present in adulthood, and it is by this route that bacteria are presumed to enter the disc. Again, the diagnosis may be difficult. Fever is not an invariable accompaniment; and in fact, may be present in only about fifty percent of patients with childhood discitis. The primary complaint may not be back pain; but, rather abdominal or leg pain. Infants may only demonstrate irritability (Table 9). A careful examination will demonstrate spinal tenderness, splinting and occasionally signs of meningeal irritation. The sedimentation rate will be elevated. Plain radiographs may show nothing initially, but, after several weeks disc space narrowing will become evident (Smith, 1933; Spiegel, 1972; Wegner, 1978) (for a full description refer to Chap. 12) (Table 10).

The adult form of discitis is almost always iatrogenic. In the past iatrogenic discitis was most often postoperative (Thibodeau, 1966), recent experi-

Table 9. Discitis in childhood. Clinical symptoms and signs

Irritable
Refusal to walk
Back pain
Abdominal pain
Hip pain

Table 10. Radiographic appearance of discitis in childhood

Disc space narrowing
End plate irregularity
Rare abscess
May fuse

Table 11. Discitis of adults

Clinical
    Insidious onset usually–rarely acute
    Severe back pain beginning weeks or months after procedure (radiographic findings
        much as in the children)

Physical findings
    Local tenderness and spasm
    Unusual neurologic findings

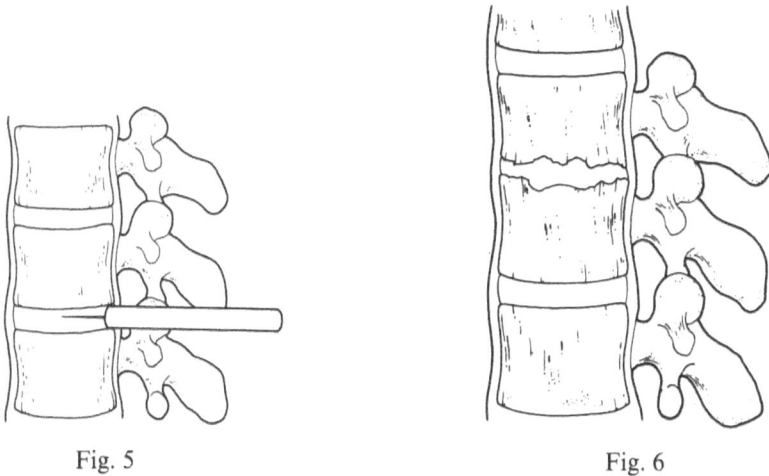

Fig. 5   Fig. 6

Fig. 5. Discitis. Aspiration and/or biopsy for attempted culture

Fig. 6. Discitis. Erosions (these are somewhat larger than average)

ence is that now they are more frequently due to innoculation during various injection procedures such as caudal block for delivery discography and chemonucleolysis (Fraser, 1986). The delay in diagnosis in these cases is often significant and in our experience was often one year or more. The patients present with severe back pain and splinting which began from one to three months following the invasive procedure and did not respond to extensive

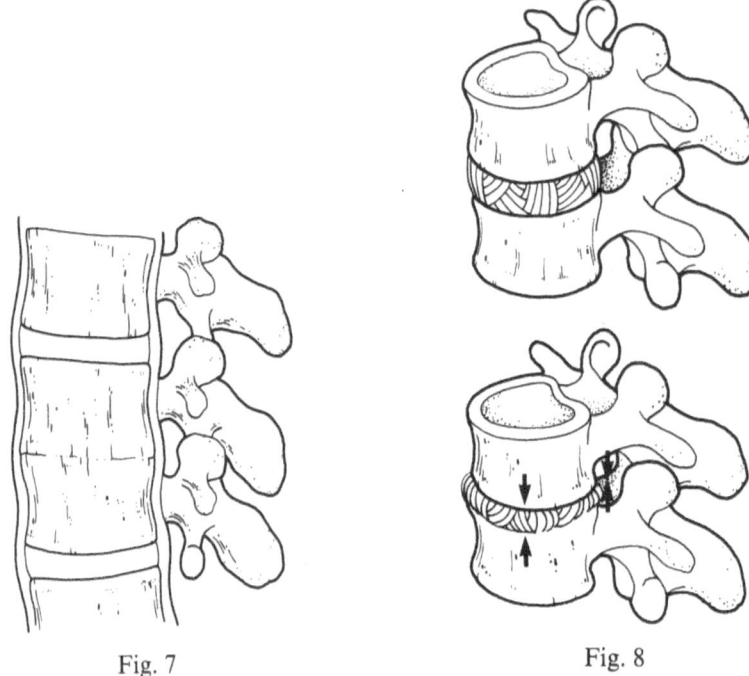

Fig. 7   Fig. 8

Fig. 7. Discitis. Autofusion

Fig. 8. Discitis. Secondary neuroforamenal stenosis

"conservative" therapy (Table 11). Positive cultures were not always obtained, but when present two organisms predominate *S. epidermidis* and *P.
acne* (Fig. 5). The number of organisms found are few and the physician is
always tempted to ignore these cultures as being "contaminated". In an
experimental study of discitis, Fraser et al. (1986) have demonstrated that
after three months the organisms cannot be found in sheep in spite of progressive destruction of disc. Further, they noted that the disc destruction
occurred only in those animals in which the live bacteria were inoculated and
not in the controls that had sterile injections. Experience on humans is
analogous. Bone scan, sedimentation rate, and magnetic resonance imaging
are helpful in the diagnosis of adult discitis. However, the sine qua non for
diagnosis remains tomography with demonstration of disc narrowing and
endplate erosions (Fig. 6).

The treatment of adult discitis is the same as that for osteomyelitis. Again,
the secret to good therapy is a timely and accurate diagnosis. After adequate
immobilization and antibiotic therapy healing with solid anterior bony fusion may occur (Fig. 7). Discitis may result in severe disc narrowing with
secondary obliteration of the neuroforamena (Fig. 8). This subluxation of the
superior facet of the lower vertebra can cause nerve root injury requiring
surgical decompression.

16 The patient with inflammatory spine disease

Sero-negative spondylarthropathies

The syndrome described in Table 1 is caused by a group of inflammatory diseases which are thought to result from a derangement of the immune mechanism of the body. These so-called sero-negative spondylarthropathies share a variety of clinical, radiographic and genetic features (Kohler and Vaughan, 1982; Moll, 1974; Brewerton et al. 1973; Jayson, 1986). Although, both inflammatory arthritis and spondylitis are major components of each of these diseases, they are not to be thought of as variations of rheumatoid arthritis. This clinical distinction is important since complications, response to therapy and progress are quite different. Inflammatory spinal disease, extra-articular foci, particularly eye disease, and a tendency for onset in young, mainly male, adults are uniting features linking this group of diseases together. Additionally, three of the five subgroups in this category have a very high incidence of the histocompatibility antigen HLA-B27 among those afflicted with the spinal component of the disease, and an even greater proportion are HLA-B27 positive if they manifest both the eye and spinal components (Table 2). The five sub-groups to be considered are: (1) ankylosing spondylitis; (2) "reactive arthritis"; (3) Reiter's syndrome; (4) inflammatory bowel disease; and (5) psoriasis (Table 3). In the inflammatory bowel disease and psoriasis the HLA-B27 antigen is not a factor unless there is spinal involvement and then not nearly in as great a proportion as in the other three groups (Mills et al., 1975).

Table 1. Symptoms and signs in patients with inflammatory spine disease

Symptoms	Signs
Chronic pain	Decreased chest expansion
Gradual onset	SI-joint stress test positive
Morning stiffness	Sero-negative
Improvement with exercise	HLA-B27 positive
Age less than 40	Late severe rigidity/deformity

Table 2. HLA association with sero-negative spondylarthropathies

Disease	HLA-B27 %
Ankylosing spondylitis	90
Reiter's syndrome	60–75
Psoriasis cutaneous	normal
peripheral arthritis	normal
axial arthritis	50
Colitic arthritis	normal
peripheral	normal
axial	50
Normal Whites	6–8
Normal Am. Blacks	2–3

Table 3. Differential diagnosis of sero-negative spondylarthropathies

	Ankylosing spondylitis	Reiter's syndrome	Inflammatory bowel disease	Psoriasis
Sacroiliitis	100% early symmetric	20% late asymmetric	20% symmetric	20% late asymmetric
Peripheral arthritis	hips and shoulders	lower extremity	hips and shoulders	upper extremity
Calcaneous periostitis	frequent	very frequent	occurs	no
Extraarticular	occurs	frequent (eye/skin)	occurs	frequent (skin)
Sex	M > F	M > F	F = M	F > M
Age at onset	≥ 20	> 20	any	any
Onset	gradual	sudden	variable	spine gradual

Ankylosing spondylitis

The most typical disease of the category is ankylosing spondylitis (Bechterew-Marie-Strümpell disease) (AS). AS is a disease which is more often detected in young males with a reported male to female ratio of 7:1 in which low back pain and stiffness are the initial complaints and may be the only symptoms for many years (Bluestone, 1985; Kohler and Vaughan, 1982). It is now believed that the true male to female ratio is closer to one to one, but that the disease is milder in the female patients, and therefore often undetected. Its prevalence is highest among white (0.1–0.2%), less common in American blacks and rare among Japanese. The stiffness and pain is often episodic and the severity of the spinal involvement is quite variable. Pain often occurs in the early morning hours, and stiffness lessens at the end of the day. Pain and stiffness increase with inactivity and improve with exercise. When the disease becomes progressive the spinal involvement moves from the sacroiliac joints upward along the spine with the cervical spine being involved last. Joints other than those of the axial skeleton can also be involved with an inflammatory arthritis and synovitis which is seldom as destructive as that of rheumatoid arthritis. In the limbs, as in the axial skeleton, progressive stiffness leading to bony ankylosis is the hallmark of this disease. The hips, shoulders and knees are the most commonly and most severely affected of the extremity joints. The peripheral arthritis is often monoarticular. In its end stage AS is easily recognized, but at the onset, which is insidious, there is often a dirth of clinical evidence obscuring the true nature of the disease. An unfortunate number of these patients are undiagnosed for a long time and some have undergone surgical procedures before the correct diagnosis is made.

The pathologic changes in AS consist of chronic inflammatory involvement of fibrocartilage, cartilage, ligaments, periosteum, adjacent bone, and sometimes of the extraskeletal fibrous tissue (Cruickshank, 1975; Schmorl and Junghans, 1971; Fassbender, 1986). At first there is an infiltration of the subchondral bone by granulation tissue causing the adjacent cartilage to be distorted and producing a very irregular surface. When synovium is the affected tissue, there is an infiltration by macrophages and lymphocytes. This is followed by replacement of the cartilage or fibrous tissue by a scar like fibroblastic invasion which rapidly ossifies. The inflammatory response in the bone adjacent to the involved fibrocartilage, ligament or periosteum is frequently quite severe. AS of the spine can resemble an infectious discitis when the spine is initially involved and, thus, can be an additional source of confusion for the treating physician.

Since the disease process is one of inflammation of fibrous tissue, bone, and cartilage, it is not surprising that organs other than joints also can become involved. Painful inflammation of the attachments of tendons and ligaments to bone (enthesopathy) occurs in the more florid cases. Eye disease occurs in about twenty-five percent of the patients as either iridocyclitis or conjunctivitis. Vascular, cardiac, and pulmonary involvement is seen in about ten percent of the patients. HLA-B27 is present in 85 to 90 percent of the patients with ankylosing spondylitis.

"Reactive arthritis"

This is a condition in which an inflammatory arthritis occurs following an intestinal infection with *Yersinia enterocolitica, Shigella flexneri, Salmonella thyphimurium,* and *Campylobacter jejuni.* Ninety percent of patients with reactive arthritis are HLA-B27 positive.

Reiter's syndrome

Reiter's syndrome consists of the triad of conjunctivitis, urethritis, and arthritis (Sharp, 1985). It is a sterile arthritis but follows either a venereal infection (non-gonococcal urethritis, cervicitis, lymphogranuloma venerium) caused by either *Chylamydia trachomatis* or Mycoplasma, or an enteric infection caused by the same organisms that cause "reactive arthritis". In fact, Reiter's syndrome is sometimes referred to as a reactive arthritis. Again the HLA-B27 association is very high (60–75%). Reiter's disease affects mainly young adults with a very strong male predilection (9:1). The diagnostic features which lead one to the probable diagnosis of Reiter's syndrome include: (1) onset within a month of urethritis or enteritis; (2) fever; (3) pauciarticular arthritis; (4) sacroiliitis; (5) skin lesions of the palms and soles; and (6) inflammation of the eye (conjunctivitis). Reiter's arthritis typically affects knees, ankles and feet. It can be quite intense, requireing exclusion of gonococcal or other pyogenic processes. Although low back pain is common, radiographic evidence of sacroiliitis is present in 20% only. Sacroiliac involvement is most frequent, and often unilateral.

Inflammatory bowel disease

Arthritis involving the peripheral joints occurs in twenty percent of patients who have inflammatory bowel disease (Ulcerative colitis, regional enteritis, and Whipple's disease). Spinal involvement occurs in five to ten percent of these patients with colitic arthritis. The HLA-B27 antigen is present in fifty percent of those with spinal involvement, but is not more commonly present in patients without spinal involvement than in the population at large. Sacroiliitis is the most frequent spinal presentation. It is indistinguishable from AS radiographically and clinically.

Psoriasis

This is a common hereditary disease of the skin affecting more than one percent of the U.S. population. Five percent of patients with proven psoriasis have an associated ankylosing spondylitis. The skin disease usually precedes the arthritis. The spinal involvement in psoriasis is subtly different than that of ankylosing spondylitis in that there is less stiffness and pain and less frequent involvement of the sacroiliac joints (Habif, 1985). Spinal involvement is more often present in males who tend to be older than the mean age of patients with psoriasis. Eye and peripheral joint disease is more common in these patients than is spinal involvement. The disease is usually slowly progressive, and not infrequently asymptomatic. The incidence of the HLA-B27 antigen is not increased in patients with skin involvement only, but is present in about 50 percent of those with spinal involvement (Bennett, 1985).

Rheumatoid arthritis

Synovial involvement of the spinal articulations occuring in patients with *rheumatoid arthritis* is, most often, a late manifestation. However, the above described diseases are not types or subgroups of rheumatoid arthritis and should not be thought of as such.

History

The history of a gradual onset of morning stiffness which improves with activity, and of early morning pain, in a patient who is less than forty years of age should alert the examining physician to the possibility of there being an inflammatory cause for the patient's complaint of lower back pain. The patient should be questioned about the possible association of previous genital or gastrointestinal infection and psoriasis. A previous history of conjunctivitis, iritis or enteropathy should also arouse suspicion of the possibility of an inflammatory cause for the lower back pain. The listing of diseases in Table 1 is a summary of the associated conditions which should be considered in detailed system review for patients with seronegative spondyloarthropathy.

Physical examination

The examination of the back in patients with seronegative spondyloarthropathy will reveal a more uniform pattern of stiffness than is commonly found in those with mechanical lower back pain. The flexion and lateral bending will be equally decreased; whereas, in the mechanical group the deficiency is more often greater in flexion than in lateral bending. The sacroiliac stress tests are often positive early on in these patients, even before there is significant spinal stiffness. Restriction of chest expansion is an important sign. Heel tenderness, tenderness in the costochondral articulations, tendonitis, and peripheral arthritis all suggest inflammatous disease. The presence of genital and oral ulcers, psoriasis, aseptic pustular lesions on the hands and feet should direct one's attention to the possibility of psoriatic arthritis or Reiter's disease. In early AS, the physical examination as well as radiographs can be normal.

Investigations

The details of the appropriate studies will be found in Chap. 2. The basic studies should consist of radiographs of the sacroiliac joints and involved portions of the spine, serum testing for the HLA-B27 antigen, and possibly a Te-99 diphosphonate bone scan. The erythrocyte sedimentation rate (ESR) is usually somewhat elevated, but may be completely normal even in severe systemic disease. The rheumatoid factor is uniformly absent except in the rare instance of the co-existence of both diseases. A positive HLA-B27 supports the likelihood of AS, while a negative result virtually excludes it. CT scans of the sacroiliac joints are much more diagnostic than standard films.

Treatment

Details of the various treatment modalities will be found in Chap. 3. In these patients the judicial use of non-steroidal anti-inflammatory drugs and exercise to maintain mobility provide the back bone of therapy.

Therapy should include (and begin with) appropriate patient education, since treatment is primarily symptomatic and the disease chronic. Corticosteroids are not very effective and should be avoided. Intra-articular injections can sometimes be helpful, however, should be used sparingly. Rheumatologic consults are often indicated.

Exercises include primarily extension treatment, pulmonary exercises and range of motions exercises. In addition, postural advice is required to prevent spinal flexion deformities.

Prognosis in AS is good. The first 10 years of disease usually predict the remainder, since severe disease mostly occurs early.

17 The patient with metabolic bone disease and low back pain

Introduction

In metabolic bone disease it is not only the bones of the vertebral column that are involved, but indeed all osseous structures throughout the body. Not infrequently, however, patients with metabolic bone disease present with back pain as their first complaint. At times symptoms are unspecific. Other times there are distinct features in the patient's presentation that lead you to believe that a metabolic bone disease may be the cause of the patient's problem. Those include extreme pain following a trivial trauma to the back, progressive kyphosis and/or scoliosis and previous distal radius and hip fractures (Table 1). Metabolic bone disease should always be suspected in elderly women with unspecific complaints and normal objective findings.

When metabolic bone disease is suspected several different tests may be done to further evaluate the patient. While some of the methods of measuring bone mineral content have been reviewed in Chap. 2, Table 2 can serve as a guideline for which additional diagnostic studies should be performed and in which order.

Table 1. Signs and symptoms of patients with metabolic disease and low back pain

Presenting complaints	Physical findings
Severe back pain after trivial trauma	Elderly white women
Progressive kyphosis and/or scoliosis	Deformity
Previous hip and/or distal radius fracture	Local tenderness
Muscular weakness and cramps	
Vague localized pain	
Renal stones	

Osteoporosis

Osteoporosis is defined as a loss of absolute bone mass with normal ratio of the bone's mineral and osteoid content. It is the result of bone resorption in excess of bone formation. The process leading to osteoporosis begins at

Table 2. Diagnostic studies in metabolic bone disease

Stage 1	Plain film radiographs
	CBC
	ESR
	Calcium
	Phosphate
	Alkaline phosphatase
Stage 2	Bone mineral density measurement
	Parathyroid hormone assay
	T3-level
	Corticoid level
	Protein electrophoresis
Stage 3	Bone biopsy

about age 30 and progresses with age. It has been estimated that males lose between 5–8% bone mass per decade, while females tend to lose 10–15%. Due to accelerated bone loss particularly subsequent to menopause one-third of all white women develop clinically significant osteoporosis. The progressive bone loss affects primarily trabecular bone and therefore is most pronounced in the vertebral bodies, the femoral necks and the metaphyses of long bones. About 25% of white women at age 75 will have a vertebral compression fracture. The actual cause of osteoporosis is unknown. What is known, however, is that the rate of bone loss is influenced by metabolic factors, immobilization, physical activity, estrogen deficiency and various endocrinopathies (Table 3). Osteoporosis is a major problem in society causing an estimated 1.3 million fractures in the U.S. yearly.

Table 3. Factors associated with an increased risk of osteoporosis

Age
Female sex
White race
Early menopause
Poor nutrition
Cigarette smoking
Inactivity
Corticosteroid medication

Clinical signs and symptoms

Back pain is the most frequent presenting complaint of patients with osteoporosis. Examination in the early stages of osteoporosis is unremarkable,

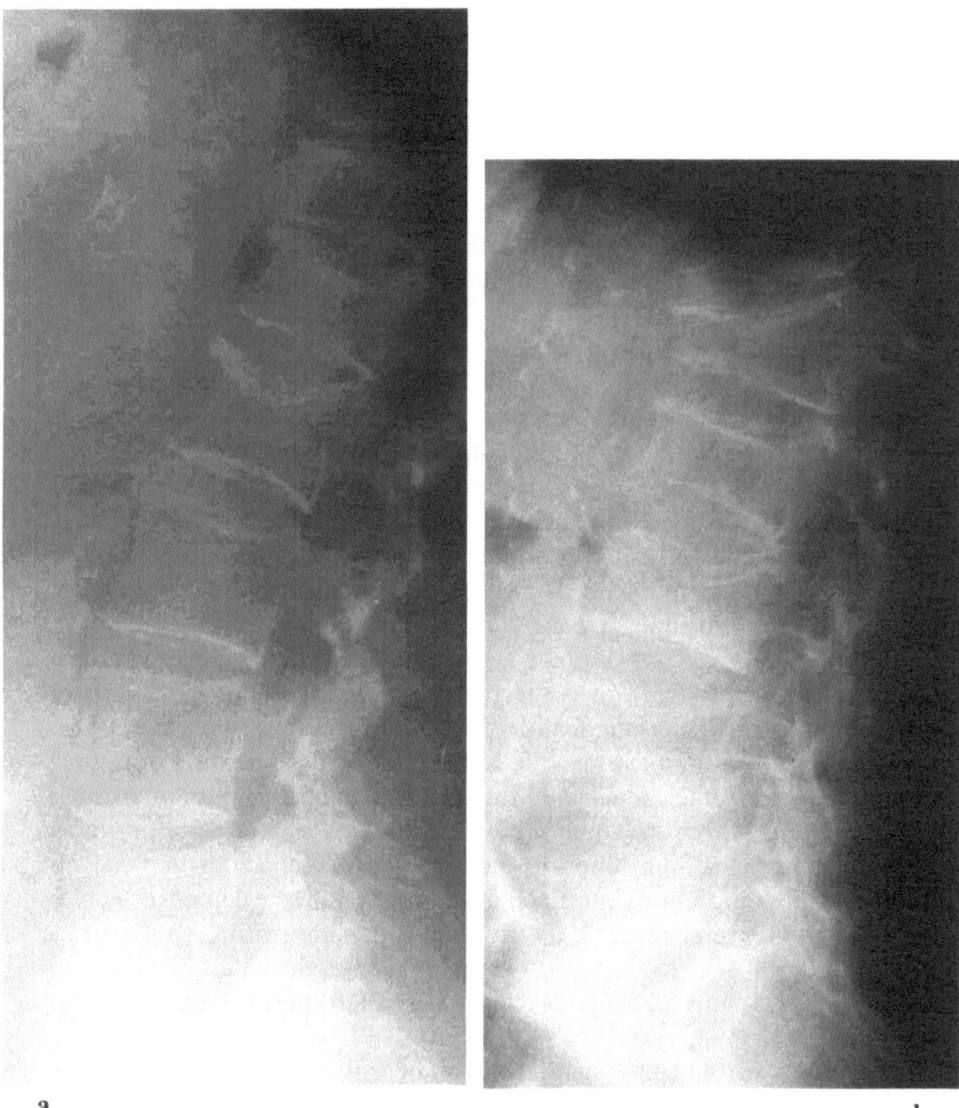

a   b

Fig. 1 a, b. Severe osteoporosis with multiple compression fractures

but with progressive disease deformity of the spine occurs often referred to as the "dowager's hump". Radiographs will not infrequently show compression fractures with a lateral projection being the most helpful (Fig. 1). About 30% of bone mineral must be lost before an increase in radiolucency can be appreciated from a plain film radiograph. Therefore, a compression fracture can be the first sign. While the compression fracture can have a different appearance, the most common is one of anterior wedging, that is the anterior aspect of the vertebral body has reduced height compared to the posterior.

The location of these vertebral fractures within the spine is quite variable. Although the fracture can be substantial, as determined from the radiograph osteoporosis rarely gives rise to sciatica and there is rarely any nerve compression involved.

There are no specific laboratory findings to make a positive diagnosis of osteoporosis. Osteoporosis, therefore, is a diagnosis of exclusion. Diseases to exclude include osteomalacia, multiple myeloma, hyperparathyroidism, hyperthyroidism and Cushing's disease. Histomorphometry based on a bone biopsy can sometimes give a positive diagnosis, but is expensive and somewhat inaccessible.

Treatment

Prophylaxis is the most important treatment method for osteoporosis. It includes dietary counseling with an emphasis on adequacy in the intake of calcium. There is no indication that excessive doses of calcium, over and above the daily dietary requirements, are beneficial. Thus in premenopausal women 1000 mg/day is sufficient, while post menopause and during pregnancy 1500 mg/day is recommended. The daily requirement for men is 1000 mg. Higher doses of calcium increase the risk of kidney stones with doubtful positive values. Exercises and an active life style should be encouraged. Estrogen replacement therapy is effective in preventing osteoporosis in women. It is indicated when a surgically induced menopause exists, while controversy exists in healthy post-menopausal women. This is because of the risk of breast and endometrial cancer. Treatment of the existing osteoporosis is still unproven. Current treatment recommendations include calcium supplement, vitamin D, sodium fluoride and estrogen. Other newer therapies include administration of calcitonin and diphosphonates to depress osteoclastic activity. Our preference is to treat these patients with 1 to 1.5 gm of calcium a day. The addition of 50–75 mg of sodium fluoride a day is attractive. However, many patients develop gastrointestinal problems and joint stiffness.

Treatment of the spine manifestations of osteoporosis is symptomatic. Pain is usually quite severe during the acute fracture episode requiring bedrest and analgesics. Sometimes pain is severe enough to require hospitalization, but often the patient can be treated at home. Corsets are helpful, while rigid metal braces can be a problem in many of these patients because of discomfort. Osteoporotic fractures heal quite readily given time but new fractures can occur. Between fractures the patient should be advised on exercises such as walking, swimming, and biking.

Osteomalacia

Osteomalacia is quite different from osteoporosis in that the ratio of mineral to osteoid is decreased. This is because in osteomalacia there is a failure of calcification of the bone matrix. While there are several causes of osteomalacia, they can usually be divided into one of five classes (Table 4). The most common causes are abnormalities in the vitamin D metabolism or a decrease in calcium absorption from the gastrointestinal tract.

Osteomalacia can present itself in many different ways clinically. Muscular weakness and vague localized pains are common along with muscle cramps. Spinal deformity can become very prominent and is usually accompanied by pain. Radiographically the vertebral bodies demonstrate biconcavity referred to as "codfish vertebra". Because of the lack of bone mineral, bone is soft but not brittle. Fractures, therefore, do not present themselves as in osteoporosis. Pseudofractures can occur and usually then are localized to the ribs and pelvic rami. They are called "Looser zones" and "milkman's fractures" and present as transverse radiolucencies, arising spontaneously. Laboratory data in osteomalacia include a lower than normal serum calcium level, slightly lower phosphate level and a mildly elevated alkaline phosphatase level. None of these values may be strikingly abnormal. Diagnosis, therefore, should be made using a bone biopsy with the specimen usually obtained from the iliac crest. The biopsy will reveal an increase in the width of the osteoid seams.

Treatment

Treatment depends on the underlying disorder. In classic osteomalacia treatment consists of 1.5 gms of calcium per day and 50,000 of vitamin D twice per week. Symptomatic treatment of the spinal condition with rest and a corset may be required.

Table 4. Causes of osteomalacia

Deficiency states	Vitamin D
	Calcium
	Phosphate
GI absorbtion defects	GI abnormality
	Biliary disease
	Absorbtion disease
Renal	
Secondary osteomalacia	Fibrous dysplasia
	Neurofibromatosis
	Soft tissue and bone neoplasm
	Anticonvulsive medication

Hyperparathyroidism

Hyperparathyroidism is an increase in the secretion of parathyroid hormone. Primary hyperparathyroidism is caused by a disease in the parathyroid glands. A single adenoma is responsible in about 80% of patients, with clear cell hyperplasia responsible for an additional 15% and cancer for 5%. Secondary hyperparathyroidism on the other hand is caused by a disorder outside the glands, usually a calcium deficiency. This triggers a release of parathyroid hormone. As parathyroid hormone is released an increasing volume calcium is reabsorbed from bone resulting in loss in bone mineral and strength.

Hyperparathyroidism occurs most often in women between their third and fifth decade of life. The onset is slow with loss of appetite, nausea, vomiting and polydipsea. Recurrent renal stones is an associated problem. The spine may or may not be affected. If so back pain and increasing kyphosis are the main presenting symptoms. In severe cases a loss of height may occur because of severe vertebral body collapse. The lateral view of the spine will show vertebral compression and wedging. Because of endplate sclerosis the picture commonly referred to as Rugger jersey spine can occur. As the disease progresses anterior wedging can increase significantly. Laboratory tests will show an increase in alkaline phosphatase, in serum calcium and a decrease in serum phosphorus level. The combination of back pain, renal stones, and abdominal pain (bones, stones, and abdominal groans) should lead to a suspicion and then the diagnosis will be confirmed using the laboratory tests.

Treatment

In primary hyperparathyroidism surgical intervention is the treatment of choice. In secondary hyperparathyroidism, on the other hand, the underlying cause should first be addressed. When calcium levels in serum return to normal the disease usually reverses.

Paget's disease

Paget's disease is a bone disease of unknown etiology which presents itself initially as a disease of excessive resorption of bone and then subsequently presents with excessive bone formation. Three phases can be distinguished in which the first is an osteolytic or destructive phase, the second a mixed stage in which bone formation and resorption occur at the same time. The final stage is the sclerotic or osteoblastic stage. All these stages can occur at the same time in the same bone. Metabolically, there is an increase in bone

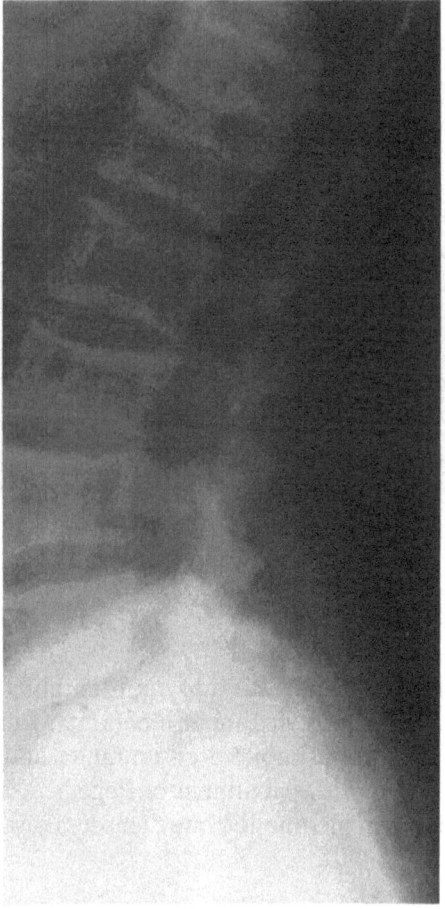

Fig. 2. Paget's disease with widespread changes

turnover with normal serum levels of calcium and phosphorus. Alkaline phosphatases are increased due to osteoblastic activity.

The spine is a common site of Paget's disease which can be painful although in most patients it does not result in pain. Dorsal kyphosis can also occur as can neurologic compression. The latter is usually due to spinal stenosis. Radiographically the lateral X-rays are the most informative as with the other metabolic bone disorders. The vertebral body is expanded and its cortex is tickened (Figs. 2 and 3). Different degrees of sclerosis occur depending on which stage the disease is in.

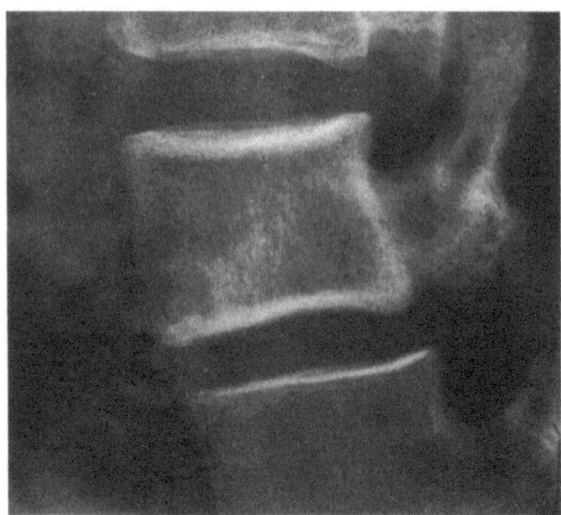

Fig. 3. Paget's disease of L3. Note the thick endplates and the course trabeculae (Pictureframe appearance)

Treatment

Most patients with Paget's disease have no symptoms and thus do not require treatment. If symptomatic, local treatment including wide laminectomy can be required. Calcitonin, diphosphonate compounds and mithramycin are three agents currently used in the treatment of Paget's disease, which should be handled by a specialist in metabolic bone disorders or an endocrinologist.

References

1 Introduction

Adams MA, Hutton HC (1985) Gradual disc prolapse. Spine 10: 524–531

Andersson GBJ (1981) Epidemiologic aspects on low back pain in industry. Spine 6: 53–60

Andersson GBJ (1982) Measurements of loads on the lumbar spine. In: White AA, Gordon SL (eds) Symposium on idiopathic low back pain. Mosby, St. Louis, pp 220–251

Andersson GBJ, Örtengren R, Nachemson A, Elfstrom G (1974) Lumbar disc pressure and myoelectric back muscle activity during sitting. Scand J Rehabil Med 6: 104–114

Andersson GBJ, Örtengren R, Herberts P (1977) Quantitaive electromyographic studies of back muscle activity related to posture and loading. Orthop Clin North Am 8: 85–96

Andersson GBJ, Murphy RW, Örtengren R, Nachemson A (1978) The influence of backrest inclination and lumbar support on the lumbar lordosis in sitting. Spine 4: 52–58

Andersson GBJ, Svensson H-O, Oden A (1983) The intensity of work recovery in low back pain. Spine 8: 880–884

Andrae R (1929) Über Knorpelknötchen am hinteren Ende der Wirbelbandscheiben im Bereich des Spinalkanals. Beitr Pathol Anat 82: 464

Biering-Sorensen F (1982) Low back trouble in a general population of 30-, 40-, 50-, and 60-year old men and women. Dan Med Bull 29: 289–299

Biering-Sorensen F (1983) A prospective study of low back pain in a general population. I. Occurrence, recurrence and etiology. Scand J Rehabil Med 15: 71–79

Chaffin DB, Andersson GBJ (1984) Occupational biomechanics. Wiley Interscience, New York

Chapman CR, Bonica JJ (1983) Current concepts: acute pain. Upjohn Publications, Kalamazoo, MI

Engel GL (1983) Pain. In: Blacklow RS (ed) MacBryde's signs and symptoms, 6th edn. Lippincott, Philadelphia, pp 41–60

Farfan HF (1973) Mechanical disorders of the low back. Lea and Fabiger, Philadelphia

Farfan HF (1984) The torsional injury to the lumbar spine. Spine 9: 53

Fine J (1985) Your guide to coping with back pain. McClelland and Stewart, Toronto

Frymoyer JW (1988) Back pain and sciatica. N Engl J Med 318: 291–300

Frymoyer JW, Pope MH, Costanza MC, Rosen JC, Goggin JE, Wilder DG (1980) Epidemiologic studies of low-back pain. Spine 5: 419–423

Frymoyer JW, Donaghy RM (1985) The ruptured intervertebral disc. Follow-up report on the first case fifty years after recognition of the syndrome and its surgical significance. J Bone Joint Surg [Am] 67: 1113–1116

Ghormley RK (1933) Low back pain with special reference to the articular facets. With presentation of an operative procedure. JAMA 101: 1773–1777

Goldthwait JE (1911) The lumbo-sacral articulation: an explanation of many cases of "lumbago", sciatica, and paraplegia. Med Surg J (Boston) 164: 355–372

Gracier KL, Holbrook TL, Kelsey J, Stauffer RN (1984) The frequency of occurrence, impact and cost of musculoskeletal conditions in the United States. Am Acad Orthop Surg, Park Ridge, IL

Hirsch C, Schajowicz F (1952) Studies on structural changes in the lumbar annulus fibrosus. Acta Orthop Scand 22: 184–231

Kellgren JH (1938) Observations on referred pain arising from muscle. Clin Sci 3: 175

Kellgren JH (1939) On the distribution of pain arising from deep somatic structures with charts of segmental pain areas. Clin Sci 4: 35

Luschka HV (1858) Die Halbgelenke des menschlichen Körpers. Reimer, Berlin

Maciewicz R, Sandrew BB (1985) Physiology of pain. In: Evaluation and treatment of chronic pain. Urban and Schwartzenberg, Baltimore Munich

Macintosh JE, Bogduk N (1987) The morphology of the lumbar erector spinae. Spine 12: 658–668

Melzak R, Wall PD (1965) Pain mechanisms. A new theory. Science 154: 971–979

Middleton ER, Teacher JH (1911) Extruded disc at the T12-L1 level. Microscopic examination showed it to be nucleus pulposus. Med J (Glasgow) 76: 1

Mixter WJ, Barr JS (1934) Rupture of the intervertebral disc with involvement of the spinal canal. N Engl J Med 211: 210–215

Mooney V, Robertson J (1976) The facet syndrome. Clin Orthop 115:149–156

Nachemson A (1960) Lumbar intradiscal pressures. Acta Orthop Scand [Suppl] 43: 1–104

Nachemson A (1981) Disc pressure measurement. Spine 6: 93–97

National Institute for Occupational Safety and Health (1981) A work practices guide for manual lifting. Tech. Report No. 81–122, U.S. Dept. of Health and Human Services (NIOSH), Cincinnati, OH

Pope MH, Wilder D, Booth J (1982) The biomechanics of low back pain. In: White AA, Gordon SL (eds) Symposium on idiopathic low back pain. Mosby, St. Louis, MO, pp 252–295

Pope MH, Frymoyer J, Andersson GBJ (1984) Occupational low back pain. Praeger Press, New York

Rees WES (1971) Multiple bilateral subcutaneous rhizolysis of segmental nerves in the treatment of intervertebral disc syndrome. Ann Gen Pract 26: 126–127

Schultz AB (1982) Mechanical factors in the etiology of idiopathic low back disorders. In: White AA, Gordon SL (eds) Symposium on idiopathic low back pain. Mosby, St. Louis, MO, pp 201–219

Shealy CN (1974) Facets in back and sciatic pain: a new approach to major pain syndromes. Minn Med 57: 199–203

Snook SH (1987) Unpublished data. Liberty Mutual Insurance Company, Hopkinton, MA

Snyder SH (1986) Drugs and the brain. Scientific American Books, New York

Spangfort EV (1972) The lumbar disc herniation: a computer aided analysis of 2504 operations. Acta Orthop Scand [Suppl] 42: 1–95

Spengler DM, Bigos SJ, Martin NA, Zeh J, Fisher L, Nachemson A (1986) Back injuries an industry: a retrospective study. I. Overview and cost analysis. Spine 11: 241–245

Svensson H-O, Andersson GBJ (1982) Low back pain in forty to forty seven year old men. I. Frequency of occurrence and impact on medical services. Scand J Rehabil Med 14: 47–53

Svensson H-O, Andersson GBJ, Johansson S, Wilhelmsson C, Vedin A (1988) A retrospective cross-sectional study of low back pain in 38–64 year old women. Spine 13: 548–552

Valkenburg HA, Haanen HCM (1982) The epidemiology of low back pain. In: White AA, Gordon SL (eds) Symposium on idiopathic low back pain. Mosby, St. Louis, MO, pp 9–22

Vernon-Roberts B (1987) Pathology of intervertebral discs and apophyseal joints. In: Jayson MI (ed) The lumbar spine and back pain. Churchill Livingstone, Edinburgh, pp 37–55

Vernon-Roberts B, Pirie CJ (1977) Degenerative changes in the intervertebral disc of the lumbar spine and their sequelae. Rheumatol Rehabil 16: 13–21

Virchow R (1858) Untersuchungen über die Entwicklung der Schädelgrunden. Reimer, Berlin

Wadell G (1987) A new clinical model for the treatment of low back pain. Spine 12: 632–644

White AA, Panjabi MM (1978) Clinical biomechanics of the spine. Lippincott, Philadelphia

Wood PHN, Badley EM (1980) Epidemiology of back pain. In: Jayson MI (ed) The lumbar spine and back pain. Pitman, London, pp 13–17

3 Treatment modalities

Ahlgren SA, Hansen T (1978) The use of lumbosacral corsets prescribed for low back pain. Prosthet Orthot Int 2: 101–104

Andersson GBJ, Schultz A, Nachemson A (1983) Intervertebral disc pressures during traction. Scand J Rehabil Med 9: 88–91

Buerger AA, Greenman PE (1985) Empirical approaches to the validation of spinal manipulation. Thomas, Springfield, OH

Deyo RA (1983) Conservative therapy for low back pain. Distinguishing useful from useless therapy. JAMA 250: 1057–1062

Deyo RA, Diehl AK, Rosenthal M (1986) How much bedrest for acute low back pain? N Engl J Med 315: 1064–1070

Dixon GW (1985) The current status of the scientific basis for manipulation. Curr Concepts Rehabil 2: 41–43

Ejeskär A, Nachemson A, Herberts P et al (1983) Surgery versus chemonucleolyis for herniated lumbar discs. Clin Orthop 174: 236–242

Ghormley RK (1983) Low back pain with special reference to the articular facets with presentation of an operative procedure. JAMA C1: 1773

Gibson T, Harkness J, Blagrave P, Graham R, Woo P, Hills R (1985) Controlled comparison of short-wave diathermy treatment with osteopathic treatment in nonspecific low back pain. Lancet: 1258–1260

Graham R (1980) Clinical trials in low back pain. Clin Rheum Dis 6: 143–157

Hadler NM, Curtis P, Gillings DB, Stinnett S (1987) A benefit of spinal manipulation as adjunctive therapy for acute low back pain: a stratified controlled trial. Spine 12: 703–706

Kane W (1977) Early detection of scoliosis. Orthopedic Digest 5: 13–17

Kendall PH, Jenkins JM (1968) Exercises for backache: a double blind controlled trial. Physiotherapy 54: 154–157

Kendall PH, Jenkins JM (1968) Lumbar isometric flexion exercises. Physiotherapy 54: 158–163

Larsson U, Chöler U, Lidström A, Lind G, Nachemson A, Nilsson B, Roslund J (1980) Auto traction for treatment of lumbago-sciatica. A multicentre controlled investigation. Acta Orthop Scand 51: 791–798

Ljunggren AE, Weber H, Larsen S (1984) Autotraction versus manual traction in patients with prolapsed lumbar intervertebral discs. Scan J Rehabil Med 16: 117–124

McCulloch JA (1977) Chemonucleolysis. J Bone Joint Surg [Br] 59: 45–52

McCulloch JA (1980) Chemonucleolysis. Experience with 2000 cases. Clin Orthop 146: 128–135

McKenzie RA (1981) The lumbar spine: mechanical diagnosis and therapy. Waikanae, New Zealand

Mayer T (1985) Using physical measurement to assess low back pain. J Musculoskeletal Med 6: 44–59

Mooney V, Robertson J (1976) The facet syndrome. Clin Orthop 115: 149–156

Nachemson AL, Elfstrom G (1970) Intravital dynamic pressure measurements in lumbar discs. Scad J Rehabil Med [Suppl] 1: 1–40

Nachemson AL (1983) Work for all: for those with low back pain as well. Clin Orthop 179: 77–85

Nachemson AL, Schultz AB, Andersson GBJ (1983) Mechanical effectiveness of lumbar spine orthoses. Scand J Rehabil Med 9: 139–149

Nordby EJ (1983) Current concepts review. Chymopapain in intradiscal therapy. J Bone Joint Surg [Am] 65: 1350–1353

Postacchini F, Lami R, Massobrio M (1987) Chemonucleolysis versus surgery in lumbar disc herniations. Spine 12: 87–96

Rees WS (1974) Multiple bilateral subcutaneous rhizolysis of segmental nerves in the treatment of intervertebral disc syndrome. Ann Gen Pract 26: 126

Rothman RH, Simeone FA (1982) The spine. WB Saunders, Philadelphia

Shealy CN (1976) Facet denervation in the management of back and sciatic pain. Clin Orthop 115: 157–164

Spitzer WO et al (1987) Scientific approach to the assessment and management of activity related spinal disorders. Spine 12 [Suppl 1]: S1–S59

Waddell G (1987) A new clinical model for the treatment of low back pain. Spine 12: 632–644

Ward NG (1986) Tricyclic antidepressants for chronic low back pain. Spine 11: 661–665

Watkins RG, Collis JS, Jr (1987) Lumbar discectomy and laminectomy. Principles and techniques in spinal surgery. Aspen, Frederick, MD

Weber H, Burton K (1986) Rational treatment of low back trouble? Clin Biomech 1: 160–167

White AH, Rothman RH, Ray CD (1987) Lumbar spine surgery: techniques and complications. C V Mosby, St. Louis, MO

Weinstein J, Spratt KF, Lehmann T, McNeill T, Hejna W (1986) Lumbar disc herniation. A comparison of the results of chemonucleolysis and open discectomy after 10 years. J Bone Joint Surg [Am] 68: 43–54

Wiesel SW, Cuckler JM, DeLuca F et al (1980) Acute low back pain: an objective analysis of conservative therapy. Spine 5: 324–330

Williams CP (1965) The lumbosacral spine. McGraw Hill, New York

4 The patient with acute low back pain

Chöler U, Larsson R, Nachemson A, Peterson L-E (1985) Back pain – attempt at a structured treatment program for patients with low back pain. Spri Report 188. Spri, Stockholm (in Swedish)

Deyo RA, Diehl AK, Rosenthal M (1986) How much bed rest for acute low back pain? N Engl J Med 315: 1064–1070

Nutter P (1987) Aerobic exercise in the treatment and prevention of low back pain. In: Deyo RA (ed) State of the art reviews: spine (occupational back pain), vol 2. Hanley and Belfus, Philadelphia, pp 137–146

Wiesel SW, Cuckler JM, DeLuca C et al (1980) Acute low back pain: an objective analysis of conservative therapy. Spine 5: 324–330

5 The patient with recurrent low back pain

Bergquist-Ullman M, Larsson U (1977) Acute low back pain in industry. A controlled prospective study with special reference to therapy and confounding factors. Acta Orthop Scand [Suppl] 170: 1–117

Biering-Sorensen F (1983) The prognostic value of the low back history and physical measurements. Doctoral Dissertation, University of Copenhagen, Denmark

Troup JDG, Martin JW, Lloyd DCEF (1981) Back pain in industry. A prospective survey. Spine 6: 61–69

6 The patient with pain radiating down the leg

Bell GR, Rothman RH (1984) The conservative treatment of sciatica. Spine 9: 54–56

Cuckler JM, Bernini PA, Wiesel SW, Booth RE, Rothman RH, Pickens GT (1985) The use of epidural steroids in the treatment of lumbar radicular pain: A prospective randomized, double-blind study. J Bone Joint Surg [Am] 67: 63–66

Dilke TFW, Burry HC, Grahame R (1973) Extradural corticosteroid injection in management of lumbar nerve root compression. Br Med J 2: 635–637

Fraser RD (1984) Chymopapain for the treatment of intervertebral disc herniation: the final report of a double-blind study. Spine 9: 815–818

Frymoyer JW (1988) Back pain and sciatica. N Engl J Med 318: 291–300

Hakelius A (1970) Prognosis in sciatica: a clinical follow-up of surgical and non-surgical treatment. Acta Orthop Scand [Suppl] 129: 1–76

Hirsch C, Nachemson A (1963) The reliability of lumbar disc surgery. Clin Orthop 29: 189–194

Kahanovitz N (1986) Presented at the Am Acad Orthop Surg, Las Vegas, NV

McCulloch JA (1980) Chemonucleolysis: experience with 2000 cases. Clin Orthop 146: 128–135

McNeill TW, Sinkora G, Leavitt F (1987) Psychologic classification of low back pain patients: a prognostic tool. Spine 12: 955–959

Postacchini I, Lami R, Massobrio M (1987) Chemonucleolysis versus surgery in lumbar disc herniation: correlation of the results to preoperative clinical pattern and size of the herniation. Spine 12: 87–96

Spangfort EV (1972) The lumbar disc herniation. A computer aided analysis of 2504 operations. Acta Orthop Scand [Suppl] 142: 1–95

Weber H (1978) Lumbar disc herniation: a prospective study of prognostic factors including a *controlled trial*. Part 1. J Oslo City Hosp 28: 33–61

Weber H (1983) Lumbar disc herniation: a controlled prospective study with ten years of observation. Spine 8: 131–140

Weinstein J, Spratt KF, Lehmann T, McNeill TW, Hejna W (1986) Lumbar disc herniation: a comparison of the results of chemonucleolysis and open discectomy after ten years. J Bone Joint Surg [Am] 68: 43–54

8 The patient with lower back pain, sciatia, and inability to void

Aho AJ, Auranen A, Pesonen K (1969) Analysis of cauda equina symptoms in patients with lumbar disc prolapse. Acta Chir Scand 135: 413–420

Floman Y, Wiesel SW, Rothman RH (1980) Cauda equina syndrome presenting as a herniated lumbar disc. Clin Orthop 147: 234–237

Peyser E, Harari A (1977) Intradural rupture of lumbar intervertebral disk. Surg Neurol 8: 95–98

Raaf J (1959) Some observations regarding 905 patients operated upon for protruded lumbar intervertebral disc. Am J Surg 97: 388–399

Shephard RH (1959) Diagnosis and prognosis of cauda equina syndrome produced by protrusion of lumbar disc. Br Med J 2: 1434–1439

Spangfort EV (1972) The lumbar disc herniation; a computer-aided analysis of 2,504 operations. Acta Orthop Scand [Suppl] 142: 1–95

Tandon PN, Sankaran B (1967) Cauda equina syndrome due to lumbar disc prolapse. Ind J Orthop 1: 112–119

Tay ECK, Chacha PB (1979) Midline prolapse of a lumbar intervertebral disc with compression of the cauda equina. J Bone Joint Surg [Br] 41: 43–46

9 The patient with lower back pain and leg pain with walking

Arnoldi CC et al (1976) Lumbar spinal stenosis and nerve root entrapment syndromes, definition and classification. Clin Orthop 115: 4

Dyck P, Doyle JP (1977) Bicycle test of Van Gelderen in the diagnosis of intermittent cauda equina compression syndrome: case report. J Neurosurg 46: 667–670

Eisenstein S (1977) The morphometry and pathologic anatomy of the lumbar spine in South African negroes and caucasoids with specific referral to spinal stenosis. J Bone Joint Surg [Br] 59: 173–180

Eisenstein S (1980) The trefoil configuration of the lumbar vertebral canal. J Bone Joint Surg [Br] 62: 73–77

Epstein JA, Epstein BS, Lavine LS (1962) Nerve root compression associated with narrowing of the lumbar spinal canal. J Neurol Neurosurg Psychiatry 25: 165–176

Kirkaldy-Willis WH (1984) The relationship of structural pathology to the nerve root. Spine 9: 49–52

Kirkaldy-Willis WH, Wedge JH, Yong Hing K, Reilly J (1978) Pathology and pathogenesis of lumbar spondylosis and stenosis. Spine 4: 319–328

Macnab I (1950) Spondylolisthesis with an intact neural arch. The so-called pseudospondylolisthesis. J Bone Joint Surg [Br] 32: 325–333

Porter RW, Hibbert C, Wellman P (1980) Back ache and the lumbar spinal canal. Spine 5: 99–105

Rothman SLG, Glenn WV (1985) Multiplanar CT of the spine. University Park Press, Baltimore, MD

Verbiest H (1954) Radicular syndromes from developmental narrowing of the lumbar vertebral canal. J Bone Joint Surg [Br] 36: 230–237

Weinstein JN, Scafuri RL, McNeill TW (1983) The Rush-Presbyterian-St. Luke's lumbar spine analysis form: a prospective study of patients with "spinal stenosis". Spine 8: 891–896

10 The patient with chronic low back pain

Addison RG (1984) Chronic pain syndrome. Am J Med 77: 54–58

Addison RG (1985) Chronic low back pain. Clin J Pain 1: 50–59

Bonica JJ, Chapman CR (1986) Biology, pathophysiology, and therapy of chronic pain. In: Berger PA, Keith H, Brodie M (eds) American handbook of psychiatry, vol 8. Basic Books, New York, pp 711–761

Cassel E (1982) The nature of suffering and the goals of medicine. N Engl J Med 306: 11: 639–645

Crock HV (1986) Internal disc disruption: a challenge to disc prolapse fifty years on. Spine 11: 650–653

Fordyce WE (1976) Behavioural methods in chronic pain and illness. CV Mosby, St. Louis, MO

Frymoyer JW, Selby DK (1985) Segmental instability: rationale for treatment. Spine 10: 280–286

Loeser JD (1982) Concepts of pain. In: Stanton-Hicks M, Boas R (eds) Chronic low
    back pain. Raven Press, New York, pp 145–148
Loeser JD, Black RG (1975) Taxonomy of pain. Pain 1: 81–84
Mayer TG, Gatchel RJ, Kishino N et al (1986) A prospective short-term study of
    chronic low back pain patients utilizing novel objective functional measurement.
    Pain 25: 53–68
Mooney V, Robertson J (1976) The facet syndrome. Clin Orthop 115: 149–156
Waddell G (1987) A new clinical model for the treatment of low-back pain. Spine
    12: 632–644
Waddell G, Main CJ, Morris EW, DiPaola M, Gray ICM (1984) Chronic low back
    pain, psychological distress and illness behaviour. Spine 9: 209–213

11 The adult patient with spine deformity and low back pain

Bosworth D, Fielding JW, Demarest L, Bonaquist M (1955) Spondylolisthesis –
    a critical review of conservative series of cases treated by arthrodesis. J Bone Joint
    Surg [Am] 37: 767
Bradford DS, Moe JH, Winter RB, Montalva FJ (1975) Scheuermann's kyphosis.
    Results of surgical treatment by posterior spine arthrodesis in 22 patients. J Bone
    Joint Surg [Am] 57: 439
Bradford DS, Brown DM, Moe JH, Winter RB, Jowsey J (1976) Scheuermann's
    kyphosis: a form of osteoporosis? Clin Orthop 118: 10
Bradford DS, Ahmed KB, Moe JH, Winter RB, Lonstein JE (1980) The surgical
    management of patients with Scheuermann's disease. A review of 24 patients
    managed by combined anterior and posterior spine fusion. J Bone Joint Surg [Am]
    62: 705–712
Jackson RP, Simmons EH, Stripinis D (1983) Incidence and severity of back pain in
    adult idiopathic scoliosis. Spine 8: 749–756
Kostuick J (1979) Decision-making in adult scoliosis. Spine 4: 521–525
Laurent LE (1958) Spondylolisthesis. Acta Orthop Scand [Suppl] 35: 1–45
Lusskin R (1965) Pain patterns in spondylolisthesis. A correlation of symptoms, local
    pathology and therapy. Clin Orthop 40: 123–136
Nachemson A (1968) A long term follow-up study of non-treated scoliosis. Acta
    Orthop Scand 39: 466–476
Ogilvie JW, Sherman J (1987) Spondylolysis in Scheuermann's disease. Spine
    12: 251–256
Rosenberg NJ (1976) Degenerative spondylolisthesis. Clin Orthop 117: 112–120
Simmons EH, Jackson RP (1979) The management of nerve root entrapment syn-
    dromes associated with collapsing scoliosis of idiopathic lumbar and thoraco
    lumbar curves. Spine 4: 533–541
Swank S, Lonstein J, Moe J, Winter R, Bradford D (1981) Surgical treatment of adult
    scoliosis: a review of 222 cases. J Bone Joint Surg [Am] 63: 268
VanDam BE, Bradford DS, Lonstein JE, Moe JH, Ogilvie JW, Winter RB (1987)
    Adult idiopathic scoliosis treated by posterior spinal fusion and Harrington
    instrumentation. Spine 12: 32–36

Weinstein SL (1986) Idiopathic scoliosis, natural history. Spine 11: 780–783

Wiltse L (1962) The etiology of spondylolisthesis. J Bone Joint Surg [Am] 44: 539–569

Wiltse L (1977) Spondylolisthesis and its treatment: conservative treatment; fusion, with and without reduction. In: Ruge D, Wiltse L (eds) Spinal disorders – diagnosis and treatment. Lea and Febiger. Philadelphia, pp 193–217

Winter RB, Moe JH, Wang JF (1973) Congenital kyphosis, its natural history and treatment as observed in a study of 130 patients. J Bone Joint Surg [Am] 56: 27–39

12 Back pain in children

Baker DR, McHollick W (1956) Spondylolysis and spondylolisthesis in children. J Bone Joint Surg [Am] 38: 933

Boston HD Jr, Bianco AJ Jr, Rhodes KH (1975) Infections in children. Orthop Clin North Am 6: 953–964

Bradford DS, Garcia A (1969) Herniations of the lumbar intervertebral disk in children and adolescents. JAMA 210: 2045–2051

Bradford DS, Moe J, Montalvo FJ et al (1974) Scheuermann's kyphosis and roundback deformity. J Bone Joint Surg [Am] 56: 740–758

Cassidy JT (1982) Textbook of pediatric rheumatology. Wiley, New York

Dandy DJ, Shannon JM (1971) Lumbosacral subluxation (group I spondylolisthesis). J Bone Joint Surg [BR] 53: 578–595

DeOrio JK, Bianco AJ Jr (1982) Lumbar disc excision in children and adolescents. J Bone Joint Surg [Am] 64: 991–996

Doyle JR (1960) Narrowing of the intervertebral disc space in children. Presumably an infectious lesion of the disc. J Bone Joint Surg [Am] 42: 1191–1200

Epstein JA, Epstein NE, Marc J, Rosenthal AD, Lavine LS (1984) Lumbar intervertebral disc herniation in teenage children: recognition and management of associated anomalies. Spine 9: 427–432

Fernbach D, Williams T, Donaldson M (1977) Neuroblastoma. In: Sutow W, Vietti T, Fernbach D (eds) Clinical pediatric oncology. CV Mosby, St. Louis, MO, pp 506–533

Garrido E, Humphreys RP, Hendrick EB, Hoffman HJ (1978) Lumbar disc disease in children. Neurosurgery 2: 22–26

Gilday L, Ash J, Rielley B (1977) Radionuclide skeletal survey for pediatric neoplasms. Radiology 123: 399–405

Gillespie R, Faithfull TK, Roth A, Hall JE (1973) Intraspinal anomalies in congenital scoliosis. Clin Orthop 93: 103–109

Greene TL, Hensinger RN, Hunter LY (1985) Back pain and vertebral changes simulating Scheuermann's disease. J Pediatr Orthop 5: 1–7

Hart FD (1955) Ankylosing spondylitis. A review of 184 cases. Ann Rheum Dis 14: 77

Handel SF, Twiford, TW, Reigel DH, Kaufman HH (1979) Posterior lumbar apophyseal fractures. Radiology 130: 629–633

Hilton RC, Ball J, Benn RT (1976) Vertebral end plate lesions (Schmorl's nodes) in the dorsolumbar spine. Ann Rheum Dis 35: 127–131

Hensinger RN, Lang JR, MacEwen GD (1976) Surgical management of spondylolis-thesis in children and adolescents. Spine 1: 207–216

Hood RW, Riseborough EJ, Nehme AM, Micheli LJ, Strand RD, Neuhauser EBD (1980) Disastematomyelia and structural spinal deformities. J Bone Joint Surg [Am] 62: 520–528

Jackson DW, Wiltse LL, Cirincione RJ (1976) Spondylolysis in female gymnasts. Clin Orthop 118: 68–73

Jayson MIV, Herbert CM, Barks JS (1973) Intervertebral discs: nuclear morphology and bursting pressures. Ann Rheum Dis 32: 308–315

Keim HA, Reina EG (1975) Osteoid osteoma as a cause of scoliosis. J Bone Joint Surg [Am] 57: 159–163

Keller RH (1974) Traumatic displacement of the cartilaginous vertebral rim: a sign of intervertebral disc prolapse. Radiology 110: 21–24

Kirwan EO, Hutton PAN, Pozo JL, Ransford AO (1984) Osteoid osteoma and benign osteoblastoma of the spine. J Bone Joint Surg [Br] 66: 21–26

Kleinman P, Rivelis M, Schneider R et al (1977) Juvenile ankylosing spondylitis. Radiology 125: 775

Kurihara A, Kataoka O (1980) Lumbar disc herniation in children and adolescents: a review of 70 operated cases and their minimum 5 year follow-up studies. Spine 5: 443–451

Krenz J, Troup JDG (1973) The structure of the pars interarticularis of the lower lumbar vertebrae and its relation to the etiology of spondylolysis. J Bone Joint Surg [Br] 55: 735–741

Leeson MC, Makley JT (1985) Metastatic skeletal disease in the pediatric population. J Pediat Orthop 5: 261–267

Letts M, Smallman T, Afanasiev R, Gouw G (1986) Fracture of the pars interartic-ularis in adolescent athletes: a clinical-biomechanical analysis. J Pediat Orthop 6: 40–46

Lippitt AB (1976) Fracture of the vertebral body end plate and disk protrusion causing subarachnoid block in an adolescent. Clin Orthop 116: 112–115

Lowrey JJ (1973) Dislocated lumbar vertebral epiphysis in adolescent children. Report of three cases. J Neurosurg 38: 232–234

McCartee CC Jr, Griffin PP, Byrd EB (1972) Ruptured calcified thoracic disc in a child. J Bone Joint Surg [Am] 54: 1272–1274

McMaster MD (1984) Occult intraspinal anomalies and congenital scoliosis. J Bone Joint Surg [Am] 66: 588–601

Maroteaux P (1979) Metastatic malignant tumors of the skeleton. In: Maroteaux P (ed) Bone diseases of children. JB Lippincott, Philadelphia, pp 411–420

Mehta MH, Murray RO (1977) Scoliosis provoked by painful vertebral lesions. Skeletal Radiol 1: 223–230

Melnick JC, Silverman FN (1963) Intervertebral disk calcification in childhood. Radiology 80: 399–408

Menelaus MB (1964) Discitis. An inflammation affecting the intervertebral discs in children. J Bone Joint Surg [Br] 46: 16–23

Micheli LJ (1979) Low back pain in the adolescent: differential diagnosis. Am J Sports Med 7: 362–364

Nesbit ME, Kieffer S, D'Angio GJ (1969) Reconstitution of vertebral height in histiocytosis X: a long-term follow-up. J Bone Joint Surg [Am] 51: 1360–1368

Ogden J, Ogden D (1982) Skeletal metastasis: the effect on the immature skeleton. Skeletal Radiol 9: 73–82

Peck FC (1957) A calcified thoracic intervertebral disk with herniation and spinal cord compression in a child. J Neurosurg 14: 105–109

Resnick D, Niwayama G (1978) Intravertebral disc herniations: cartilaginous (Schmorl's nodes). Radiology 126: 57–65

Schaller JG (1977) Ankylosing spondylitis of childhood onset. Arthritis Rheum 20: 398

Schechter LS, Smith A, Pearl M (1972) Intervertebral disc calcification in childhood. Am J Dis Child 123: 608–611

Scheuermann HW (1921) Kyphosis dorsalis juvenilis. Z Orthop Chir 41: 305

Sherman FC, Rosenthal RK, Hall JC (1979) Spine fusion for spondylolysis and spondylolisthesis in children. Spine 4: 59–67

Sonnabend DH, Taylor TKF, Chapman GK (1982) Intervertebral disc calcification syndromes in children. J Bone Joint Surg [Br] 64: 25–31

Sorensen HK (1964) Scheuermann's kyphosis: clinical appearances, radiography, aetiology, and prognosis. Munksgaard, Copenhagen

Spiegel PG, Kengla KW, Isaacson AS, Wilson JC Jr (1972) Intervertebral disc-space inflammation in children. J Bone Joint Surg [Am] 54: 284–296

Techakapuch S (1981) Rupture of the lumbar cartilage plate into the spinal canal in an adolescent. A case report. J Bone Joint Surg [Am] 63: 481–482

Turner RH, Bianco AJ Jr (1971) Spondylolysis and spondylolisthesis in children and teenagers. J Bone Joint Surg [Am] 53: 1298–1306

Wassmann K (1951) Kyphosis Juvenilis Scheuermann – an occupational disorder. Acta Orthop Scand 21: 65–74

Wenger DR, Bobechko WP, Gilday DL (1978) The spectrum of intervertebral disc space infection in children. J Bone Joint Surg [Am] 60: 100–108

Wiltse LL (1961) Spondylolisthesis in children. Clin Orthop 21: 156–163

Wiltse LL, Widell EH, Jackson DW (1975) Fatigue fracture: the basic lesion in isthmic spondylolisthesis. J Bone Joint Surg [Am] 57: 17–22

Winter RB, Haven JJ, Moe JH, LaGaard SM (1974) Diastematomyelia and congenital spine deformities. J Bone Joint Surg [Am] 56: 27–39

Winter RB, Lipscomb PB Jr (1978) Back pain in children. Minn Med 21: 141–147

Young J, Miller R (1975) Incidence of malignant tumors in U.S. children. J Pediatr 54: 254–258

13 The patient with functional disease/malingering

Chapman CR, Bonica JJ (1983) Current concepts: acute pain. Upjohn Publications, Kalamazoo, MI

Deyo RA, Diehl AK (1986) History predictive of low back pain disabilities. Presented at the Am Rheumatism Assoc and Arthritis Health Prof Assoc Annual Meeting, New Orleans

Engel GL (1983) Pain. In: Blacklow RS (ed) MacBryde's signs and symptoms, 6th edn. Lippincott, Philadelphia, pp 41–60

Gatchel RJ, Mayer TG, Capra P, Diamond MA, Barnett MA (1986) The utility of the Million Behavioral Health Inventory in predicting physical function in low back pain patients. Presented at the 13th Annual Meeting Int Soc Study of the Lumbar Spine, Dallas, TX

Hendler N, Mollett A, Viernstein M, Schroeder D, Rybock J, Campbell J, Levin S, Long D (1985) A comparison between the MMPI and the "Hendler Back Pain Test" for validating the complaint of chronic back pain in men. J Neurol Orthop Med Surg 6: 333–337

Leavitt F (1985) Pain and deception: use of verbal pain measurement as a diagnostic aid if differentiating between clinical and simulated low-back pain. J Psychosom Res 29: 495–505

Leavitt F, Garron DC (1979) Validity of a back pain classification scale among patients with low back pain not associated with demonstratable organic disease. J Psychosom Res 23: 301–306

Leavitt F, Sweet JJ (1986) Characteristics and frequency of malingering among patients with low back pain. Pain 25: 357–364

Maciewicz R, Sandrew BB (1985) Physiology of pain. In: Aronoff GM (ed) Evaluation and treatment of chronic pain. Urban & Schwarzenberg, Baltimore Munich, p 17ff

Melzack R (1975) The McGill pain questionnaire: major properties and scoring methods. Pain 1: 277–299

Melzack R, Wall PD (1965) Pain mechanisms: a new theory. Science 154: 971–979

McNeill TW, Sinkora G, Leavitt F (1986) Psychologic classification of low-back pain patients: a prognostic tool. Spine 11: 955–959

Snyder SH (1986) Drugs and the brain. Scientific American Library, WH Freeman and Co, New York Oxford

Smith RG, Monson RA, Ray DC (1986) Psychiatric consultation in somatization disorder: a randomized controller study. N Engl J Med 314: 1407–1413

Waddell G, Mann TS (1985) Medico-legal factors in low back pain. Abstracts of papers, Annual Meeting Int Soc Study of the Lumbar Spine, Sydney, 12: 139

Waddell G, McCulloch JA, Kummell EG, Venner RM (1980) Nonorganic physical findings in low back pain. Spine 5: 117–125

Waddell G, Main CJ, Morris EW, Di Paola M, Gray ICM (1984) Chronic low-back pain, psychologic distress, and illness behavior. Spine 9: 209–213

Ward NG (1986) Tricyclic antidepressants for chronic low-back pain. Spine 11: 661–665

Weintraub MI (1977) Hysteria: a guide to diagnosis. Clin Symp 29: 2–31

14 The patient with a spine tumor

Boland PJ, Lane JM, Sundaresan N (1987) Tumors of the lumbosacral spine. In: Camins M, O'Leary P (eds) The lumbar spine. Raven Press, New York, pp 223–244

Dahlin DC (1978) Bone tumors: general aspects and data on 6,221 cases. CC Thomas, Springfield, OH

Huvos HG (1979) Bone tumors: diagnosis, treatment, and prognosis. WB Saunders, Philadelphia

Keim HA, Reina EG (1975) Osteoid osteoma as a cause of scoliosis. J Bone Joint Surg [Am] 57: 159–166

Kirwan EO'G, Hutton PAN, Ransford AO (1984) Osteoid osteoma and benign osteoblastoma of the spine: clinical presentation and treatment. J Bone Joint Surg [Am] 66: 21–26

Mindell ER (1981) Current concepts review: chordoma. J Bone Joint Surg [Am] 63: 501–505

Ransford AO, Pozo JL, Hutton PAN, Kirwan EOG (1984) The behaviour pattern of the scoliosis associated with osteoid osteoma or osteoblastoma of the spine. J Bone Joint Surg [Br] 66: 16–20

Russin LA, Robinson MJ, Engle HA, Sonni A (1982) Ewing's sarcoma of the lumbar spine: a case report of long-term survival. Clin Orthop 164: 126–129

Schajowicz F (1981) Tumors and tumor like conditions of the bone and joints. Springer, New York Heidelberg Berlin

Shives TC, Dahlin DC, Sim FH, Pritchard DJ, Earle JD (1986) Osteosarcoma of the spine. J Bone Joint Surg [Am] 68: 660–668

Siegal T, Tiqva P, Siegal T (1985) Vertebral body resection for epidural compression by malignant tumors: results of forty-seven consecutive operative procedures. J Bone Joint Surg [Am] 67: 375–382

Sim FH, Dahlin DC, Stauffer RN, Laws ER (1977) Primary bone tumors simulating lumbar disc syndrome. Spine 2: 65–74

Simeone FA, Lawner PM (1982) Intraspinal neoplasms. In: Rothman RH, Simone FA (eds) The spine. WB Saunders, Philadelphia, pp 1041–1054

Weinstein JN, McLain RF (1987) Primary tumors of the spine. Spine 12: 843–851

15 The patient with spinal infection

Batson OC (1940) The function of vertebral veins and their role in the spread of metastasis. Ann Surg 112: 138–149

Eismont FJ et al (1983) Vertebral osteomyelitis in infants. J Bone Joint Surg [Br] 64: 32–35

Eismont FJ et al (1983) Pyogenic and fungal vertebral osteomyelitis with paralysis. J Bone Joint Surg [Am] 65: 19–29

Fraser RD et al (1986) Discitis following chemonucleolysis: an experimental study. 1986 Volvo Award in basic science. Spine 11: 679–687

Friedman B (1966) Chemotherapy of tuberculosis of the spine. J Bone Joint Surg [Am] 48: 451–473

Griffiths HED et al (1971) Pyogenic infections of the spine. J Bone Joint Surg [Br] 53: 383–391

Hodgson AR, Stock FE (1960) Anterior spine fusion for the treatment of tuberculosis of the spine. J Bone Joint Surg [Am] 42: 295–310

Hughes SPF, Fitzgerald RH (1986) Musculoskeletal infections. Year Book Medical Publishers, Chicago

Kulowski J (1936) Pyogenic osteomyelitis of the spine. J Bone Joint Surg 18: 343–364

Lifeso RM et al (1985) Tuberculous spondylitis in adults. J Bone Joint Surg [Am] 67: 1405–1413

Major RA (1948) Classic descriptions of disease. CC Thomas, Springfield, OH, pp 52–53

Medical Research Council (1978) Five-year assessments of controlled trials of ambulatory treatment and anterior spinal fusion in the management of tuberculosis of the spine: studies in Bulawayo (Rhodesia) and in Hong Kong. J Bone Joint Surg [Br] 60: 163–177

Medical Research Council (1982) A ten year assessment of a controlled trial comparing debridement and anterior spine fusion in the management of tuberculosis of the spine in patients on standard chemotherapy in Hong Kong. J Bone Joint Surg [Br] 64: 393–398

Morris E et al (1965) Localized osseous cryptococcosis. J Bone Joint Surg [Am] 47: 1027–1029

Puig-Guri J (1946) Pyogenic osteomyelitis of the spine. J Bone Joint Surg [Br] 28: 29–39

Rang M (1966) Anthology of orthopaedics. Livingstone, Edingburgh, pp 7–13

Schmorl G, Junghans H (1971) The human spine in health and disease, 2nd edn, translated by EF Besemann. Grune and Stratton, New York

Smith AD (1933) A benign form of osteomyelitis of the spine. JAMA 101: 335

Spiegel PG et al (1972) Intervertebral disc-space inflammation in children. J Bone Joint Surg [Am] 54: 284–296

Stauffer RN (1975) Pyogenic vertebral osteomyelitis. Orthop Clin North Am 6: 1015–1027

Steindler A (1929) Diseases and deformities of the spine and thorax. CV Mosby Co, St. Louis, MO

Thibodeau AA (1966) Closed space infection following removal of lumbar intervertebral disc. Clin Neurosurg 14: 337–360

Trueta J (1959) The three types of acute haematogenous osteomyelitis: a clinical and vascular study. J Bone Joint Surg [Br] 41: 671–680

Waldvogel FA et al (1970) Osteomyelitis: a review of clinical features, therapeutic considerations and unusual aspects (3 parts). N Engl J Med 282: 198–206, 260–266, 316–322

Waldvogel FA et al (1980) Osteomyelitis: the past decade. N Engl J Med 303: 360–370

Wegner DR et al (1978) Spectrum of intervertebral disc-space inflammation in children. J Bone Joint Surg [Am] 60: 100–108

Weissberg ED et al (1974) Clinical features of neonatal osteomyelitis. Pediatrics 53: 505–510

Wiley AM, Trueta J (1959) The vascular anatomy of the spine and its relationship to pyogenic vertebral osteomyelitis. J Bone Joint Surg [Br] 41: 796–809

Winter WG et al (1978) Coccidiodal spondylitis. J Bone Joint Surg [Am] 60: 240–244

16 The patient with inflammatory spine disease

Kohler PF, Vaughan J (1982) The autoimmune diseases. JAMA 248: 2646–2657

Moll JMH (1974) Association between ankylosing spondylitis, psoriatic, arthritis, Reiter's disease, the intestinal arthropathies, and Behcet's syndrome. Medicine 53: 343–364

Mills DM, Arai Y, Gupta RC (1975) HL-A antigens and sacroilitis. JAMA 231: 268–270

Cruickshank B (1975) Pathology of ankylosing spondylitis. Bull Rheum Disc 34: 87–91

Bluestone R (1985) Ankylosing spondylitis. In: McCarty DJ (ed) Arthritis and allied conditions, 10th edn. Lea and Febiger, Philadelphia, pp 819–840

Jayson MIV (1986) Spinal diseases and back pain. In: Dieppe PA et al (eds) Atlas of clinical rheumatology. Lea and Febiger, Philadelphia, pp 17.13–17.15

Brewerton DA et al (1973) Reiter's disease and HLA-B27. Lancet 2: 996–998

Schmorl G, Junghans H (1971) The human spine in health and disease, 2nd edn, translated by EF Besemann. Grune and Stratton, New York

Sharp JT (1985) Reiter's syndrome (reactive arthritis). In: McCarty DJ (ed) Arthritis and allied conditions, 10th edn. Lea and Febiger, Philadelphia, pp 841–848

Fassbender HG (1986) Joint destruction in various arthritic diseases. In: Kuettner K et al (ed) Articular cartilage biochemistry. Raven Press, New York

Habif TP (1985) Clinical dermatology. CV Mosby Co, St. Louis MO

Bennett RM (1985) Psoriatic arthritis. In: McCarty DJ (ed) Arthritis and allied conditions, 10th edn. Lea and Febiger, Philadelphia, pp 850–866

Subject index

Neuro–Orthopedics

Editor-in-Chief: H. Verbiest
Assistant Chief Editor: P. F. van Akkerveeken
and an International Editorial Board covering the fields of orthopedics, neurosurgery, biomechanics, neurology, neurophysiology, anatomy, radiology, rheumatology, rehabilitation, biochemistry, and peripheral nerves.

New in 1986, Neuro-Orthopedics takes a unique approach to disorders and injuries of the musculo-skeletal system *in conjunction with* the nervous system, and includes articles on applied research as well as diagnosis and clinical management. The journal addresses neuro-regulation as a cybernetic system controlling postural, locomotor, or other motor activities of the head, spine, shoulder, pelvic girdle, arms, and legs. Spinal disorders — their multitude of symptoms and possible strategies for treatment — are covered in Neuro-Orthopedics. Other topics include problems in rehabilitation or reconstructive surgery of tetra- or paraplegia, peripheral limb paralysis, neurovascular problems in the hand, or other forms of postural and movement disorders. Neuro-Orthopedics publishes papers on the diagnoses, causes, origins and developments of disorders, along with optimal therapeutic strategies in the following areas — orthopedics, neurosurgery, traumatology, neurology, neuroradiology, biomechanics, anatomy, clinical neurophysiology, rheumatology, and rehabilitation.

Subscription Information:
1989. Vols. 7—8 (2 issues each):
DM 224,—, öS 1560,—, plus carriage charges

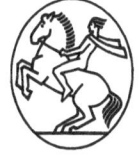

Springer-Verlag Wien New York

Moelkerbastei 5, A-1010 Wien · Heidelberger Platz 3, D-1000 Berlin 33 · 175 Fifth Avenue, New York, NY 10010, USA · 37-3, Hongo 3-chome, Bunkyo-ku, Tokyo 113, Japan

M. Bard / J.-D. Laredo (eds.)

Interventional Radiology in Bone and Joint

With a Foreword by **A. Ryckewaert**

1988. 194 figures. XII, 273 pages.
Cloth DM 292,—, öS 2050,—
ISBN 3-211-82029-9

Prices are subject to change without notice

Various sections of the book discuss:
Trephine bone and joint biopsies, including vertebral discs, sacro-iliac joints, peripheral bone, synovium, and soft tissues, using either fluoroscopic, echographic or CT guidance — Chemonucleolysis — Foraminal steroid injection for cervicobrachial nerve root pain — arthrography and selective steroid injection in the treatment of vertebral facet syndromes — Aspiration of calcium deposits of the rotator cuff tendons — steroid injection of bone cysts — vascular embolization of bone metastases and primary tumors — management of vertebral hemangiomas — new trends, such as percutaneous discectomy, with presentation of conflicting views on the utility of these techniques.
Each section includes a complete description of instruments involved, including information on manufacturers, as well as each procedure's techniques, results and indications.
This text supplies in a single volume complete information on performance of these new techniques in skeletal radiology.

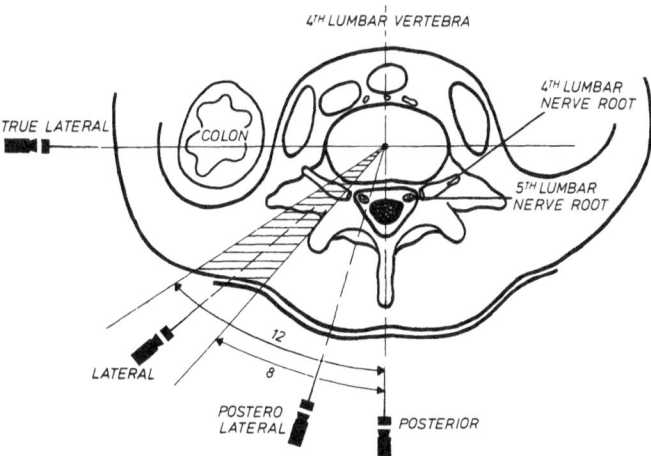

Springer-Verlag Wien New York

Moelkerbastei 5, A-1010 Wien · Heidelberger Platz 3, D-1000 Berlin 33 · 175 Fifth Avenue, New York, NY 10010, USA · 37-3, Hongo 3-chome, Bunkyo-ku, Tokyo 113, Japan

Armin K. Thron
Vascular Anatomy of the Spinal Cord

Neuroradiological Investigations and Clinical Syndromes

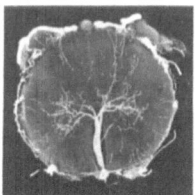

With collaboration of Ch. Rossberg
and A. Mironov

1988. 74 partly colored figures. VII, 114 pages.
Cloth DM 98,—, öS 690,—
ISBN 3-211-82015-9

The book summarizes the anatomic guidelines of external blood supply to the spinal cord. The basic principles of arterial supply and venous drainage are illustrated by explicit schemes for quick orientation.

In the first part of the book, systematic radiologic-anatomic investigations of the superficial and deep vessels of all segments of the spinal cord are introduced. The microvascular morphology is portrayed by numerous microradiographic sections in all three dimensions without overshadowing. The excellent three-dimensional representation of the vascular architecture illustrates elementary outlines and details of arterial territories, anastomotic cross-linking as well as the capillary system, particularly the hitherto unknown structure of the medullary venous system with its functionally important anastomoses and varying regional structures. These often new radiologic-anatomic findings are discussed as to their functional and pathophysiologic impact and constitute the basis on which to improve our modest understanding of vascular syndromes of the spinal cord. The neurosurgeon as well as the neuroradiologist familiar with endovascular techniques are offered information on microvascular morphology necessary for interventions at the spinal cord.

The second part of the book focuses on clinical syndromes and illustrates the present diagnostic contribution of spinal angiography with special reference to the diagnosis of spinal vascular anomalies and arteriovenous malformations. Though widely underrated in the past, the pathogenetic role of the spinal venous system in direct or indirect circulatory disorders of the spinal cord is emphasized. The book fills an obvious void both from a pathologic-anatomic and a clinical point of view, and should therefore attract every physician remotely interested in neurology.

Springer-Verlag Wien New York

Mölkerbastei 5, A-1010 Wien · Heidelberger Platz 3, D-1000 Berlin 33
175 Fifth Avenue, New York, NY 10010, USA
37-3, Hongo 3-chome, Bunkyo-ku, Tokyo 113, Japan

Serge Gracovetsky

The Spinal Engine

1988. 176 figures. XIV, 505 pages.
Cloth DM 98,—, öS 690,—. ISBN 3-211-82030-2

Prices are subject to change without notice

This book deals with the human spine with particular emphasis on the lumbar spine. It reviews the existing biomechanical theories on the function of the spine, analysing their limitations, and showing in what way they could be improved.

The human gait is traditionally believed to be the function of the legs. The book presents arguments and data that challenge that belief. It proposes that the spine is the primary engine which makes us move. This engine, inherited from our fish ancestors, was never transferred to any extremity during our long evolutionary journey.

The theory of the spinal engine is new and provoking. It positions the vertebrates as benefiting from the earth's gravitational field for their activities. The theory resolves many apparent contradictions in the experimental data collected by the scientific peers. It shows in what way everybody did hold a piece of the truth.

In short, the theory of the spinal engine represents the framework into which the pieces of an immense puzzle fit.

The spine is described as a machine subjected to the basic laws of physics. It opens a new field in robotics.

The theory enables the process of injury and repair to be understood. It provides a method for evaluating the function of the spine in clinical terms which in turn is useful in the diagnosis of a patient.

Presenting the spine in the context of the evolutionary theory contributes towards a generalization of the basic laws of life. It opens the mind to a new interpretation of known facts.

Springer-Verlag Wien New York

Moelkerbastei 5, A-1010 Wien · Heidelberger Platz 3, D-1000 Berlin 33 · 175 Fifth Avenue, New York, NY 10010, USA · 37-3, Hongo 3-chome, Bunkyo-ku, Tokyo 113, Japan